SCIENCE *of*

ANALYZE YOUR TECHNIQUE, PREVENT INJURY, REVOLUTIONIZE YOUR TRAINING

RUNNING

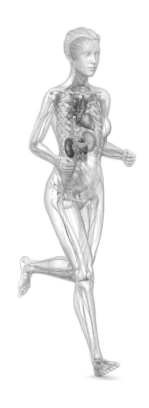

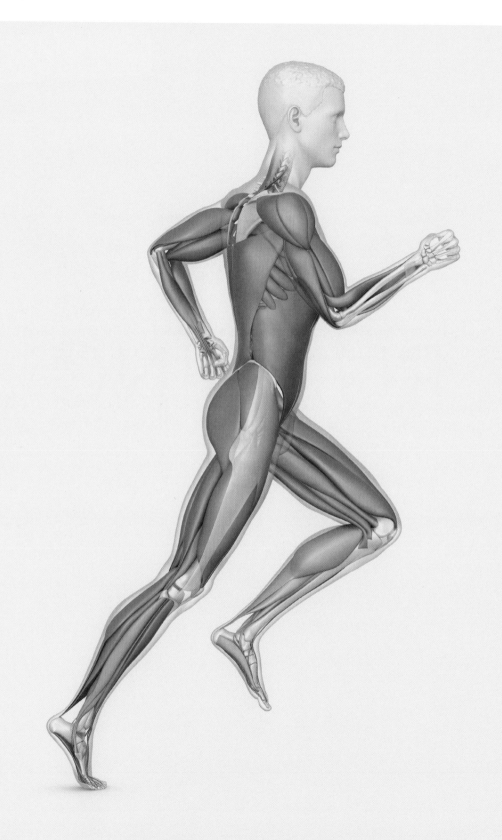

SCIENCE *of*

ANALYZE YOUR TECHNIQUE, PREVENT INJURY, REVOLUTIONIZE YOUR TRAINING

RUNNING

Chris Napier, PhD

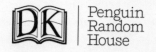

Senior Editor **Salima Hirani**
Senior Designer **Clare Joyce**
Project Editor **Shashwati Tia Sarkar**
Project Art Editor **Philip Gamble**
Editor **Megan Lea**
US Editor **Kayla Dugger**
Designer **Alison Gardner**
Editorial Assistant **Kiron Gill**
Producer, Pre-Production
David Almond
Producer **Francesca Sturiale**
Jacket Designer **Amy Cox**
Jacket Co-ordinator **Lucy Philpott**

Senior Editor **Alastair Laing**
Managing Editor **Dawn Henderson**
Managing Art Editor
Marianne Markham
Art Director **Maxine Pedliham**
Publishing Director
Mary-Clare Jerram

Illustrations **Arran Lewis**

First American Edition, 2020
Published in the United States by DK Publishing
1450 Broadway, Suite 801, New York, NY 10018

A catalog record for this book is available from
the Library of Congress.
ISBN 978-1-4654-8957-9

Printed and bound in China

A WORLD OF IDEAS:
SEE ALL THERE IS TO KNOW
www.dk.com

CONTENTS

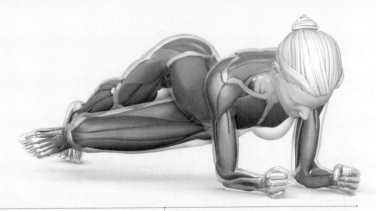

FOREWORD

Running is easy: you just put one foot in front of the other and go. So why learn the science behind it? When you scratch the surface, you find there is more to this biomechanical and physiological phenomenon than meets the eye. If your aim is to enhance performance and prevent injury, familiarizing yourself with the science of running can help you achieve your goals and take more pleasure in a sport that millions enjoy worldwide.

WHY RUN?

There are many good reasons to run, in addition to the sheer pleasure of it. Regular running is associated with many health benefits that can improve your quality of life. Running makes you stronger and healthier, and as your body becomes increasingly robust in response to this dynamic activity, you become less likely to develop disease or physical disability.

Recreational running can help prevent obesity, hypertension, type 2 diabetes, osteoarthritis, respiratory disease, and cancer and improves sleep quality. Even in low doses, running is associated with a substantial reduction in risk of death from all causes, including cardiovascular disease.

The psychological benefits of recreational running include stress relief, mood boosts, and potentially protection against depression, anxiety, and dementia. Social interaction through running groups and involvement in group events such as Parkrun also improves well-being.

While the health potentials involved are clearly considerable, running is not without its own risks. In fact, certain injuries are associated specifically with running—"runner's knee," for instance. However, there is much you can do to mitigate the risk, and that is where the science comes in.

USING THE SCIENCE

As a physical therapist, I have helped thousands of runners, from novice to elite, continue with the activity they love. My work is informed by my research into running-related injury, and I have seen time and again in my clients how an understanding of why injury occurs and how best to recover can improve their experience of running.

But the science of running can help with more than just injury prevention. If you want to improve as a runner, understanding the physiology and biomechanics involved is a game changer. Small adjustments in form can lead to big improvements if you know what to look out for and how to address it. And even a modest strength-training program can reap rewards on the roads, trails, or track if

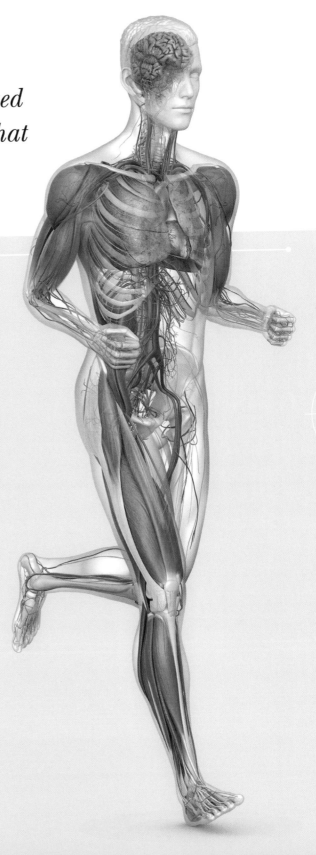

> ## *Regular running* *is associated with many* **health benefits** *that improve* **quality of life**

you know which exercises target the key muscle groups used in running.

Runners are known for having an obsession with numbers, from tracking mileage to recording personal bests, but knowing how to use the data to maximize performance is what makes the difference. Similarly, knowing how your body works allows you to use it optimally. To be a better runner, you should know which types of training make you faster, which exercises make you stronger, and which race-day strategies help you perform at your best. Jerry Ziak, my co-author on the chapter *How to Train*, is an experienced coach who has designed thousands of training programs for athletes of all levels. We hope the knowledge we share enhances your performance and training experience and helps you enjoy a lifetime of pain-free running.

Chris Napier, PT, PhD
Sport Physical Therapist
2:33 marathon PB

INTRODUCTION

When it comes to running, a little knowledge can go a long way toward enhancing performance and preventing injury. This book offers the latest research into running biomechanics alongside advice on training techniques that have been proven to work under laboratory conditions, on the track, and out on the trails.

Understanding how your body responds to running enables you to **optimize speed, strength,** *and* **performance**

ABOUT THIS BOOK

No matter what your level of ability, motivations, or goals may be, applying the science of running to your training with this book as your guide will bring you significant benefits as a runner.

Chapter 1, *Running Anatomy*, delves into the physiology of running. This will help you understand what happens within your body in order to enable you to run, as well as what your body needs to be able to do so optimally.

Chapter 2, *Preventing Injury*, explores how running-related injuries occur. It outlines measures you can take to reduce your own risk of injury or recover quickly if you do become injured—which is likely at some point.

All runners can improve their form and running experience by incorporating into their training regime some or all of the *Strength Exercises* in Chapter 3. These have been specially selected to target the most important muscle groups in running in order to make them strong enough to be able to withstand the impact and training load of endurance running. These exercises are also valuable to the injured runner looking to rehabilitate.

Chapter 4, *How to Train*, outlines all you need to know to train effectively and safely. Whether you want to learn how to design a bespoke training plan and adapt it as you progress, are looking for a race-specific plan to help you prepare for a particular event, or need a walk-run program that will take you from zero to 5K safely and quickly, this chapter provides expert guidance to help you meet those personal targets and succeed at racing.

A note on terminology

On pp.10–11, you will find illustrated definitions of the clinical terms used to describe body movements. Being able to follow these terms as you study the subject of running enables you to understand the movements involved accurately, and you can apply this understanding to your own anatomy and running gait. Knowledge of these terms will also help you to follow the instructions for the strength exercises in this book.

MYTH BUSTING

Runners quickly discover that there is plenty of contradictory advice out there. With so much conflicting information readily available, running can become a confusing subject to explore. Do not be misguided by the common myths shown here, which have all been debunked by research.

MYTH

FACT

> " "
> *Running will **hurt my knees** and result in arthritis when I am older*

HELPS PREVENT OSTEOARTHRITIS

There is growing evidence to show that recreational running can protect against the development of knee osteoarthritis. There is also evidence to suggest that even if you have osteoarthritis, running may not make it worse and could in fact improve the associated symptoms.

> " "
> *I was injured because I didn't **stretch enough** before I ran*

YOU SHOULD DO DYNAMIC STRETCHING

Research shows that static stretching does not reduce the risk of injury and can actually decrease performance. It will not assist in recovery postworkout but may improve joint flexibility and aid relaxation. Include dynamic stretching (involving movement) as part of a general warm-up (see p.76).

> " "
> *I was injured because I wore the **wrong shoes** for my foot type*

SHOE TYPE DOES NOT MATTER

Evidence is lacking to support the idea that any particular shoe type—whether minimalist, maximalist, traditional, or otherwise—can help prevent injury. Runners should, however, avoid any rapid changes in shoe type (see p.64) and monitor their overall training load (see pp.168–169) to reduce their risk of injury.

> " "
> *I should do **high-rep, low-resistance** strength training to build the muscle strength I need for running*

HIGH-RESISTANCE TRAINING IS BEST

This is a misconception. Muscular endurance is improved during running, so endurance exercises should not be the focus of resistance training. A heavy resistance-training program twice a week for 6 weeks or longer has been shown to improve running performance and reduce injury risk.

> " "
> *If I want to run faster and be injury-free, I need to **forefoot strike***

NEITHER FOOTSTRIKE PATTERN IS BETTER

The idea that a forefoot strike reduces injury risk and improves running economy compared to a rearfoot strike is false. While the type of injury may vary depending on where on your foot you land, the overall incidence of injury does not.

TERMINOLOGY GUIDE

The body's joints accommodate a range of movements, and each type of movement can be described precisely using the terms illustrated here. I use these terms throughout this book, notably in the instructions for strength exercises on pp.100–155, so mark this page for easy reference.

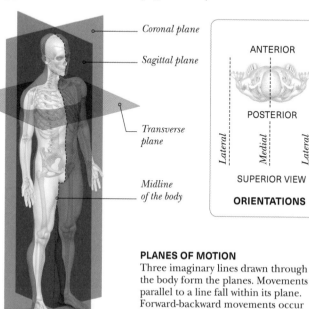

- Coronal plane
- Sagittal plane
- Transverse plane
- Midline of the body

PLANES OF MOTION

ORIENTATIONS

ANTERIOR

POSTERIOR

Lateral · Medial · Lateral

SUPERIOR VIEW

PLANES OF MOTION
Three imaginary lines drawn through the body form the planes. Movements parallel to a line fall within its plane. Forward-backward movements occur within the sagittal plane, side-to-side movements fall within the coronal or frontal plane, and rotational movements occur within the transverse plane.

Hip

Being a ball-and-socket joint (see p.21), the hip joint is capable of a large range of motion in multiple planes of movement. The hip is able to move into flexion/extension, adduction/abduction, and internal/external rotation.

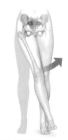

ADDUCTION
The thigh moves inward toward the midline.

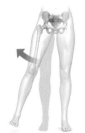

ABDUCTION
The thigh moves away from the midline.

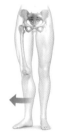

EXTERNAL ROTATION
The thigh rotates outward.

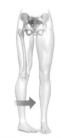

INTERNAL ROTATION
The thigh rotates inward.

Ankle and foot

There are more than 30 joints in the ankle and foot, allowing for complex and varied movements. The ankle, primarily a hinge joint (see p.20), produces dorsiflexion and plantarflexion. Eversion and inversion occur at the subtalar joint, just below the ankle. Movements such as pronation and supination are combined movements involving the foot and ankle.

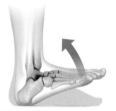

DORSIFLEXION
Bending at the ankle so that the toes point upward.

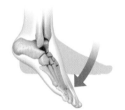

PLANTARFLEXION
Bending at the ankle so that the toes point downward.

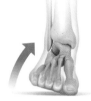

EVERSION
Turning at the ankle so that the sole of the foot faces outward.

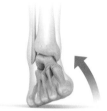

INVERSION
Turning at the ankle so that the sole of the foot faces inward.

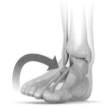

PRONATION
Combination of dorsiflexion, eversion, and abduction.

Spine

The spine provides structural support for the upper body and transfers loads between lower and upper body. It is capable of flexion, extension, rotation, side flexion, and combinations of these.

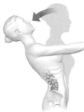 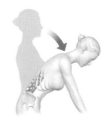

EXTENSION
Bending at the waist to move the torso backward.

FLEXION
Bending at the waist to move the torso forward.

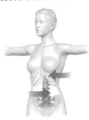 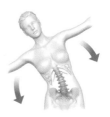

ROTATION
Turning the trunk to the right or left on the midline.

SIDE FLEXION
Bending the trunk to the right or left from the midline.

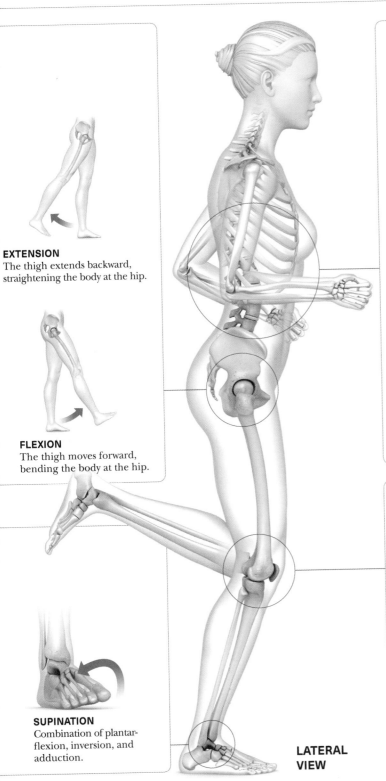

EXTENSION
The thigh extends backward, straightening the body at the hip.

FLEXION
The thigh moves forward, bending the body at the hip.

SUPINATION
Combination of plantar-flexion, inversion, and adduction.

LATERAL VIEW

Knee

The knee, primarily a modified hinge joint (see p.20), sustains loads of up to 10 times body weight during running. Flexion and extension are the main movements, although it is also capable of some abduction/adduction and internal/external rotation.

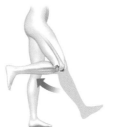 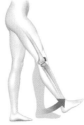

FLEXION
Bending at the knee, which decreases the joint angle.

EXTENSION
Straightening at the knee, which increases the joint angle.

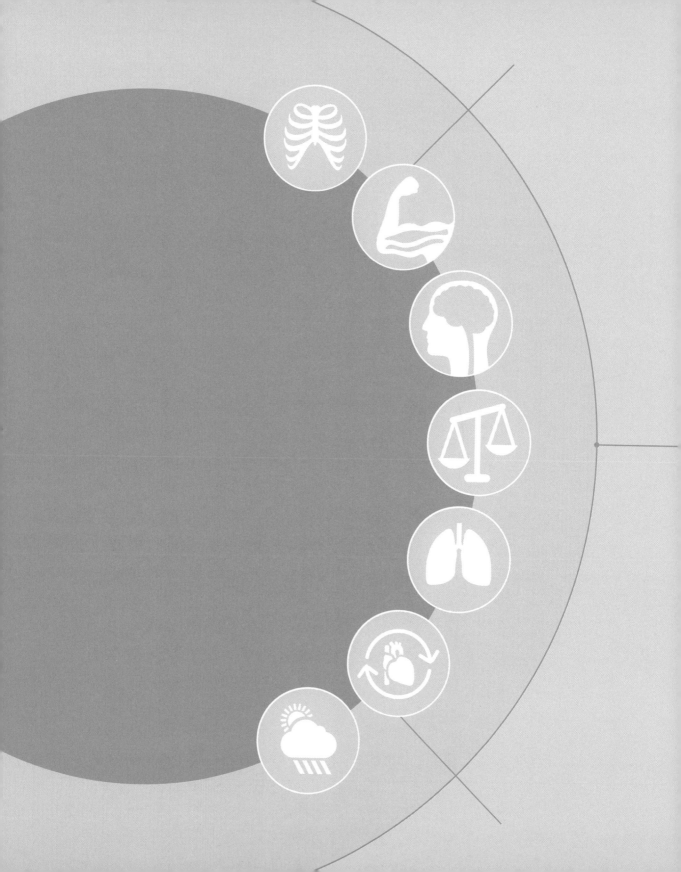

RUNNING ANATOMY

Running motion requires the body to work like a complex machine, with many functions taking place simultaneously in order to achieve this dynamic action. An understanding of the biomechanics and physiology involved can help you improve your performance and keep yourself safe and injury-free. This chapter explores the body systems that enable running and explains how they can be adapted to help you become a faster, more efficient runner.

HOW WE RUN

The simple act of putting one foot in front of the other requires the integration of muscles, joints, and the nervous system. Each component is important for optimal performance, technique, and safety, and with a little understanding of anatomy, each can be improved through training.

THE **RUNNING CYCLE**

When you run, your body combines specific joint and muscle actions to enable each leg to perform a sequence of movements in tandem with the other. This cycle is repeated thousands of times during a run. The running cycle is defined by four key events in the sequence: initial contact, midstance, toe-off, and swing. With each step, the body manages the significant ground reaction force (GRF, see pp.46–47) experienced on impact and recycles the energy into the next step.

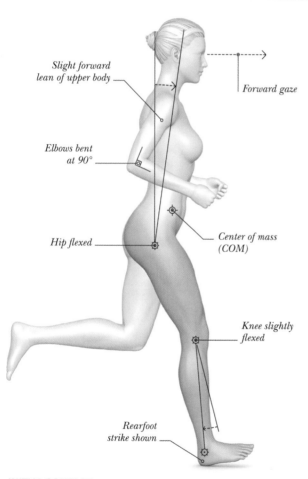

Slight forward lean of upper body

Forward gaze

Elbows bent at 90°

Hip flexed

Center of mass (COM)

Knee slightly flexed

Rearfoot strike shown

INITIAL CONTACT
Most runners land on the heel and others land on the midfoot or forefoot. Footstrike pattern (see p.72), the leg's posture at footstrike, and where the foot lands in relation to the body's center of mass (COM) all affect how the GRF is distributed through the body.

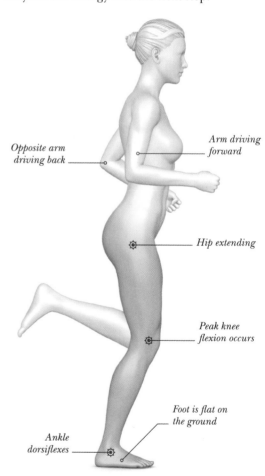

Opposite arm driving back

Arm driving forward

Hip extending

Peak knee flexion occurs

Foot is flat on the ground

Ankle dorsiflexes

MIDSTANCE
At this point, halfway between initial contact and toe-off, the vertical GRF is at its maximum, stretching muscles and tendons in the leg. The leg goes from experiencing the initial braking force to generating propulsion force. The COM is now at its lowest.

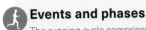

Events and phases

The running cycle comprises a sequence of moments or "events" that are grouped into two main phases—stance and swing. When a leg is in contact with the ground, it is in stance phase. This phase begins at initial contact and ends at toe-off and is made up of three subphases (see pp.66–68). Swing phase begins when the foot leaves the ground. It starts and ends with a "float" subphase, when both feet are off the ground (see p.69).

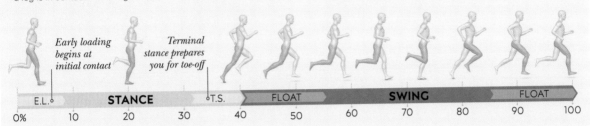

Early loading begins at initial contact

Terminal stance prepares you for toe-off

| E.L. | STANCE | T.S. | FLOAT | SWING | FLOAT |

0%   10   20   30   40   50   60   70   80   90   100

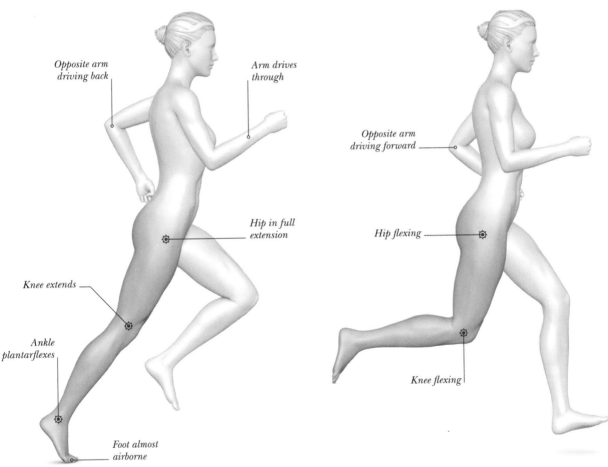

Opposite arm driving back

Arm drives through

Hip in full extension

Knee extends

Ankle plantarflexes

Foot almost airborne

Opposite arm driving forward

Hip flexing

Knee flexing

TOE-OFF
The hip and knee extend and the ankle plantarflexes to propel the body into toe-off. As the foot leaves the ground, the ankle is maximally plantarflexed and the hip and knee are maximally extended to drive the body forward.

SWING
While off the ground, the leg swings from its toe-off position behind the torso to just ahead of the COM, ready for initial contact. Most of the energy required for this movement is generated by the elastic recoil of muscles and tendons stretched during stance phase.

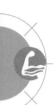

MECHANICS
OF MOVEMENT

Skeletal muscles are attached to bones by tendons. Some, such as the hamstrings, are long and cross multiple joints. Others, such as the intrinsic muscles of the foot, are short and confined to small areas.

MUSCULAR SYSTEM

Muscles create movement through thousands of forceful contractions, demonstrating endurance and resilience in response to repetitive usage. Runners need strong legs, but also strength in the core and arms to drive movement. Strength training (see pp.96–155) can improve running performance and help prevent injury.

Pectorals
Pectoralis major
Pectoralis minor

Intercostal muscles

Brachialis

Abdominals
Rectus abdominis
External abdominal obliques
Internal abdominal obliques
(deep, not shown)
Transversus abdominis

Hip flexors
Iliopsoas (iliacus and psoas major)
Rectus femoris (see quadriceps)
Sartorius
Adductors (see below)

Adductors
Adductor longus
Adductor brevis
Adductor magnus
Pectineus
Gracilis

Quadriceps
Rectus femoris
Vastus medialis
Vastus lateralis
Vastus intermedius (deep, not shown)

Ankle dorsiflexors
Tibialis anterior
Extensor digitorum longus
Extensor hallucis longus

Muscle fibers run in parallel

Elbow flexors
Biceps brachii
Brachialis (deep)
Brachioradialis

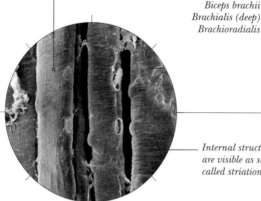

Internal structures are visible as stripes called striations

Skeletal muscle fibers
These fibers are made up of sliding micro-filaments, which contract to create movement. Training improves blood flow and nerve supply to fibers, enabling muscles to produce more power and endure longer contractions.

SUPERFICIAL

DEEP

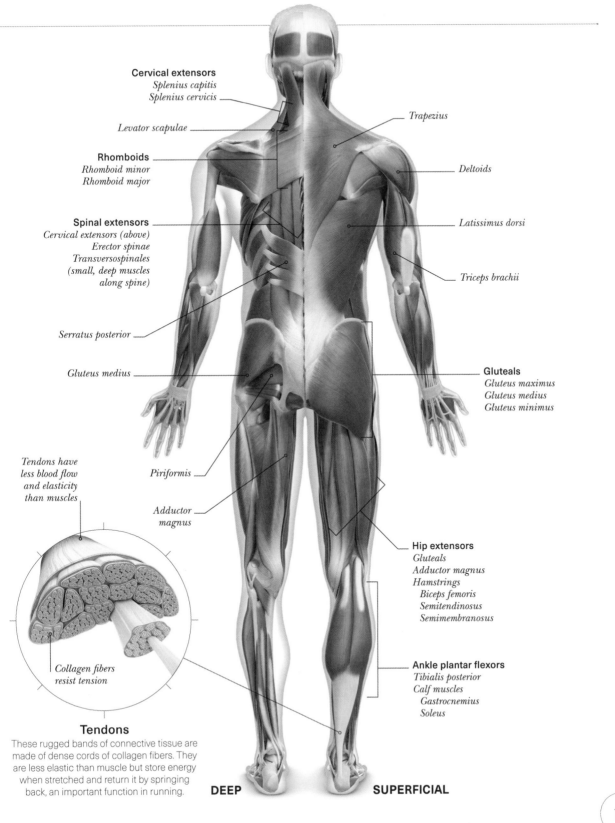

Cervical extensors
Splenius capitis
Splenius cervicis

Levator scapulae

Rhomboids
Rhomboid minor
Rhomboid major

Spinal extensors
Cervical extensors (above)
Erector spinae
Transversospinales
(small, deep muscles
along spine)

Serratus posterior

Gluteus medius

Piriformis

Adductor
magnus

Trapezius

Deltoids

Latissimus dorsi

Triceps brachii

Gluteals
Gluteus maximus
Gluteus medius
Gluteus minimus

Hip extensors
Gluteals
Adductor magnus
Hamstrings
Biceps femoris
Semitendinosus
Semimembranosus

Ankle plantar flexors
Tibialis posterior
Calf muscles
Gastrocnemius
Soleus

Tendons have
less blood flow
and elasticity
than muscles

Collagen fibers
resist tension

Tendons
These rugged bands of connective tissue are
made of dense cords of collagen fibers. They
are less elastic than muscle but store energy
when stretched and return it by springing
back, an important function in running.

DEEP

SUPERFICIAL

17

HOW MUSCLES WORK

Most of the body's muscles are skeletal muscles. They attach to the skeleton and are under voluntary control. Their fibers respond to the firings of motor neurons, which are controlled by the central nervous system (see p.38). Skeletal muscles often work in pairs that operate on either side of a joint to control the direction of movements. Nerve impulses trigger muscle fibers to pull on the bones via tendons to produce muscle movement.

Types of contraction

There are three main types of muscle contraction.
Concentric: The muscle shortens during contraction.
Eccentric: The muscle lengthens during contraction.
Isometric: The length of the muscle remains unchanged during contraction.

In running, eccentric contractions relate to the absorption and storage of ground reaction forces (GRF, see pp.46–47), while concentric contractions relate to the forward propulsion of the body.

MUSCLE KEY

- Concentric:
  Shortening
  under tension

- Eccentric:
  Lengthening
  under tension

- Lengthening
  without tension
  (stretching)

- Isometric:
  Held muscles
  without motion

ECCENTRIC CONTRACTION
The calf and quadriceps muscles engage eccentrically during the early loading phase (see p.66), lengthening as they absorb the impact force of landing. The Achilles tendon also lengthens as it absorbs GRF.

Quadriceps
contract eccentrically to absorb the GRF

Hamstrings
contract concentrically

Calf muscles
contract eccentrically to absorb the GRF

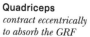

Achilles tendon
lengthens
The Achilles tendon plays an important role in running. During this stance, it lengthens under tension. Just like a stretched elastic band, this tendon stores a significant amount of GRF energy for use during the toe-off.

EARLY LOADING

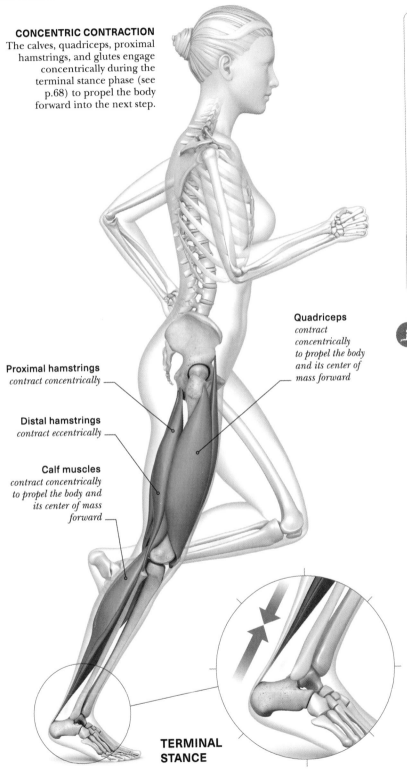

CONCENTRIC CONTRACTION
The calves, quadriceps, proximal hamstrings, and glutes engage concentrically during the terminal stance phase (see p.68) to propel the body forward into the next step.

Proximal hamstrings
contract concentrically

Distal hamstrings
contract eccentrically

Calf muscles
contract concentrically to propel the body and its center of mass forward

Quadriceps
contract concentrically to propel the body and its center of mass forward

TERMINAL STANCE

Muscle repair

Muscles are made of cylindrical cells bundled together and covered in connective tissue. Muscle damage triggers the repair process. White blood cells clear dead tissue, then new fibers and connective tissue form while new blood vessels and nerves are generated.

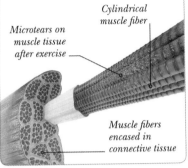

Microtears on muscle tissue after exercise

Cylindrical muscle fiber

Muscle fibers encased in connective tissue

TRAINING ADAPTATIONS

Slow- and fast-twitch muscle fibers

There are two types of skeletal muscle fiber: slow-twitch and fast-twitch. Slow-twitch fibers, being relatively resistant to fatigue, are used during steady-state aerobic exercise. Fast-twitch fibers are able to generate explosive force and activity but can only sustain this for short periods. Although training cannot change fibers from one type to the other, the kind of training you do determines which type increases in size and/or quantity within muscle.

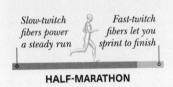

Slow-twitch fibers power a steady run

Fast-twitch fibers let you sprint to finish

HALF-MARATHON

Achilles tendon
shortens

At toe-off, the springlike Achilles tendon recoils, allowing the elastic energy stored during the loading phase to assist in propulsion.

JOINTS

Connections between bones are called joints. These can be fibrous (as in the sutures of the skull), cartilaginous (as in the pubic symphysis), or synovial (as in the knee). In synovial joints, the articulating bones are well cushioned in a fluid-filled cavity. These joints are further categorized according to their shape and structure. The types of synovial joint used most in running are gliding, hinge, and ball-and-socket joints.

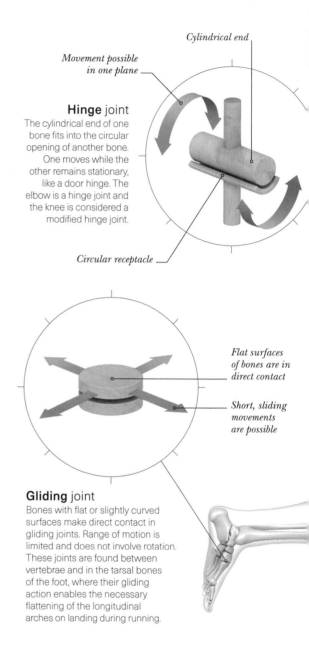

Cylindrical end

Movement possible in one plane

Hinge joint
The cylindrical end of one bone fits into the circular opening of another bone. One moves while the other remains stationary, like a door hinge. The elbow is a hinge joint and the knee is considered a modified hinge joint.

Circular receptacle

Flat surfaces of bones are in direct contact

Short, sliding movements are possible

Gliding joint
Bones with flat or slightly curved surfaces make direct contact in gliding joints. Range of motion is limited and does not involve rotation. These joints are found between vertebrae and in the tarsal bones of the foot, where their gliding action enables the necessary flattening of the longitudinal arches on landing during running.

Inside a synovial joint

Adjoining bones sit within a cavity filled with synovial fluid. This lubricates the joint, reducing friction between the bones and enabling greater movement. The bones are capped with smooth, dense cartilage, allowing them to glide across one another with minimal friction. A capsule of connective tissue surrounds the joint, supporting movement while resisting dislocation. Ligaments around and within the joint hold the bones together.

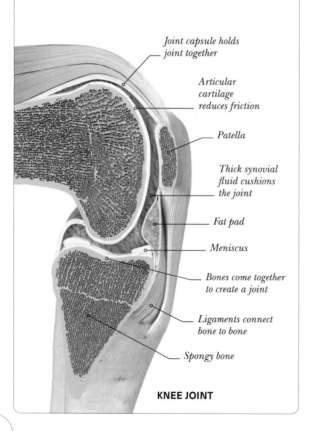

Joint capsule holds joint together

Articular cartilage reduces friction

Patella

Thick synovial fluid cushions the joint

Fat pad

Meniscus

Bones come together to create a joint

Ligaments connect bone to bone

Spongy bone

KNEE JOINT

TYPES OF SYNOVIAL JOINT
The body coordinates the actions of many joints in order to run, and the movements allowed by each type of joint dictate how the body moves while running. The shape and structure of each joint determines the range of movement it will enable.

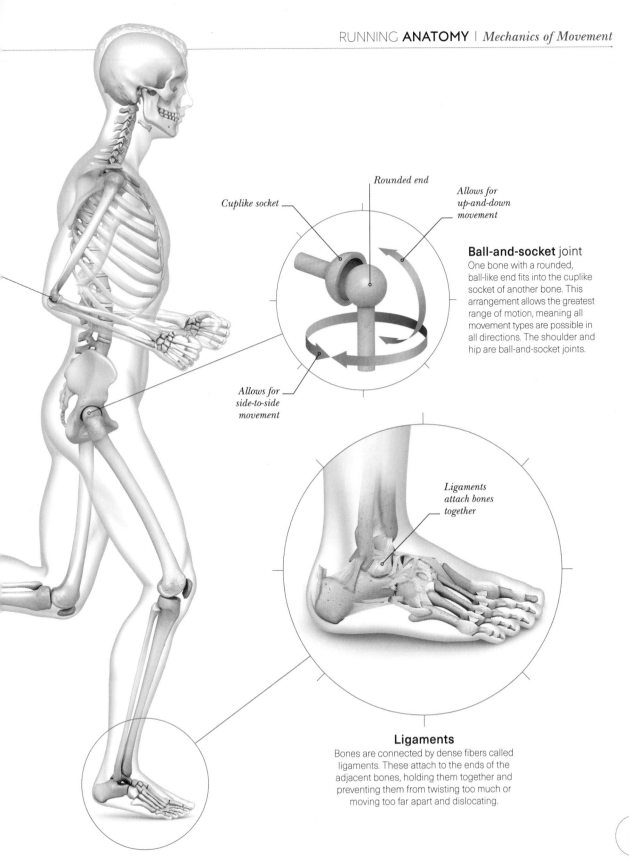

Rounded end

Cuplike socket

Allows for up-and-down movement

Ball-and-socket joint
One bone with a rounded, ball-like end fits into the cuplike socket of another bone. This arrangement allows the greatest range of motion, meaning all movement types are possible in all directions. The shoulder and hip are ball-and-socket joints.

Allows for side-to-side movement

Ligaments attach bones together

Ligaments
Bones are connected by dense fibers called ligaments. These attach to the ends of the adjacent bones, holding them together and preventing them from twisting too much or moving too far apart and dislocating.

ANKLE AND FOOT

The ankle and foot provide the foundation for every step you take. This stable base absorbs the ground reaction force (see pp.46–47) and generates strength for toe-off. The ligaments of the foot form an archlike triangular framework, which sits above a branched fibrous band spanning the sole. This unique structure allows the foot to work as both a lever—pivoting the leg during the transition from braking into accelerating—and a spring for toe-off.

Foot core

The interplay between the intrinsic and extrinsic muscles of the foot (see p.102), its tendons, and the sensory and motor nerves that control the arches provides strength and stability for each step. How these elements work together is similar to how the core stabilizes the lower back and pelvis.

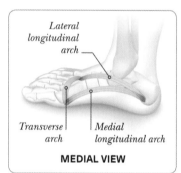

MEDIAL VIEW

Lateral longitudinal arch

Transverse arch

Medial longitudinal arch

FOOT ARCHES
The tarsal and metatarsal bones connect to form three arches, braced by ligaments, muscles, and tendons. This framework spans from the heel across to the metatarsal bones on either side of the foot, creating a stable triangular strut.

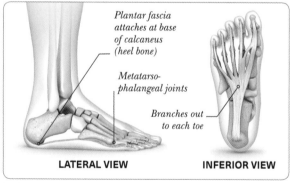

Plantar fascia attaches at base of calcaneus (heel bone)

Metatarso- phalangeal joints

Branches out to each toe

LATERAL VIEW

INFERIOR VIEW

PLANTAR FASCIA
This strong fibrous band runs across the base of the foot and branches out to each toe, constraining collapse of the medial longitudinal arch. It acts like a cable joining the calcaneus and the metatarsophalangeal joints and shortens when the toes are dorsiflexed (see p.10), stiffening the arch.

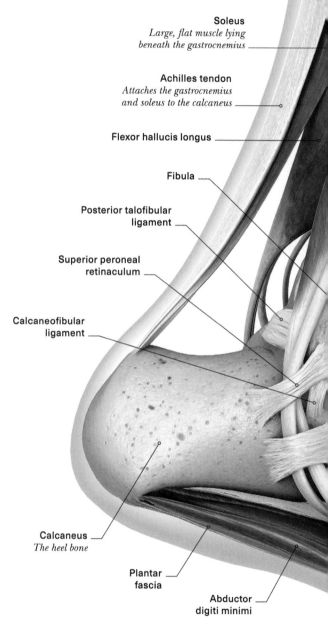

Soleus
Large, flat muscle lying beneath the gastrocnemius

Achilles tendon
Attaches the gastrocnemius and soleus to the calcaneus

Flexor hallucis longus

Fibula

Posterior talofibular ligament

Superior peroneal retinaculum

Calcaneofibular ligament

Calcaneus
The heel bone

Plantar fascia

Abductor digiti minimi

FOOT STRUCTURE
There are 3 arches; 26 bones; 33 joints; and more than a hundred muscles, tendons, and ligaments in the foot. This complex structure is regularly subjected to loads of up to three times your body weight during running.

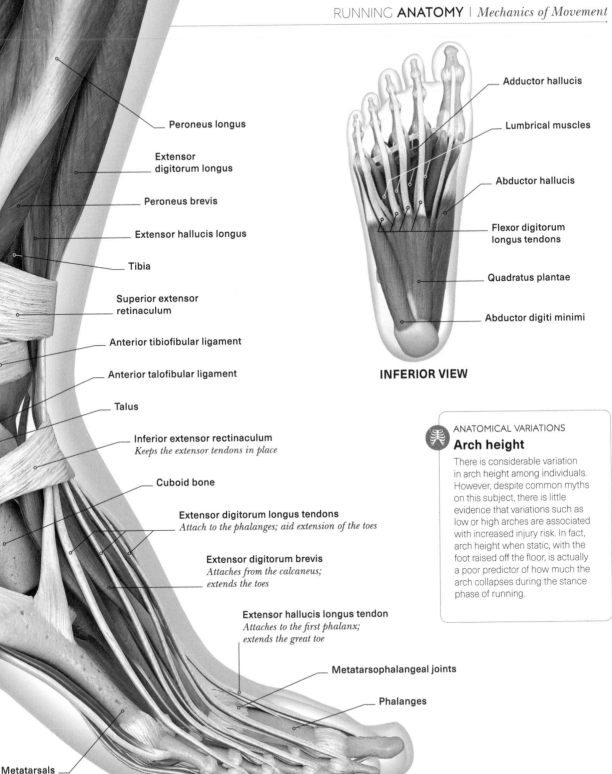

Peroneus longus

Extensor digitorum longus

Peroneus brevis

Extensor hallucis longus

Tibia

Superior extensor retinaculum

Anterior tibiofibular ligament

Anterior talofibular ligament

Talus

Inferior extensor rectinaculum
Keeps the extensor tendons in place

Cuboid bone

Extensor digitorum longus tendons
Attach to the phalanges; aid extension of the toes

Extensor digitorum brevis
Attaches from the calcaneus; extends the toes

Extensor hallucis longus tendon
Attaches to the first phalanx; extends the great toe

Metatarsophalangeal joints

Phalanges

Metatarsals

LATERAL VIEW

Adductor hallucis

Lumbrical muscles

Abductor hallucis

Flexor digitorum longus tendons

Quadratus plantae

Abductor digiti minimi

INFERIOR VIEW

ANATOMICAL VARIATIONS
Arch height
There is considerable variation in arch height among individuals. However, despite common myths on this subject, there is little evidence that variations such as low or high arches are associated with increased injury risk. In fact, arch height when static, with the foot raised off the floor, is actually a poor predictor of how much the arch collapses during the stance phase of running.

KNEE

The knee is the body's largest joint. It is the meeting point of the femur and tibia, capped by the patella. Primarily a hinge joint, the knee can perform some gliding action (see p.20) and internal and external rotation. When we run, the knee bears enormous weight (equal to 8–12 times your body weight) while providing flexible movement, making it vulnerable to injury.

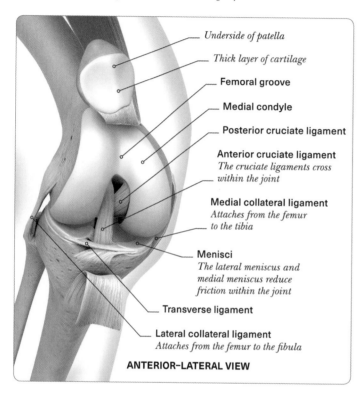

Underside of patella

Thick layer of cartilage

Femoral groove

Medial condyle

Posterior cruciate ligament

Anterior cruciate ligament
The cruciate ligaments cross within the joint

Medial collateral ligament
Attaches from the femur to the tibia

Menisci
The lateral meniscus and medial meniscus reduce friction within the joint

Transverse ligament

Lateral collateral ligament
Attaches from the femur to the fibula

ANTERIOR–LATERAL VIEW

Vastus lateralis
A large part of the quadriceps

Iliotibial band
Thick connective tissue stretching over the outer thigh

Biceps femoris (long head)

Behind the patella

The patella sits in a groove between two projections (condyles) on the femur. Most of its joint surface is covered in cartilage, which dissipates the large compression forces created during running. Impact forces or rotation can cause the patella to shift within the groove, causing patellofemoral pain. Strong ligaments crossing behind the patella help stabilize the knee from within, while ligaments on either side harness the sides of the joint.

Lateral collateral ligament
Attaches from the femur to the fibula

Fibula

Penoneus longus

Soleus

ANATOMICAL VARIATIONS

Q-angles

The Q-angle is the angle between two lines. One is drawn between the anterior superior iliac spine (ASIS) and the center of the patella and the other extends from the tibial tubercle up through the center of the patella. It ranges from 13–18°. The size of this angle has more to do with overall height than with gender or pelvic width. A larger Q-angle has been associated with an increased injury risk—and in particular, to patellofemoral pain (see p.57)—but research does not support this link.

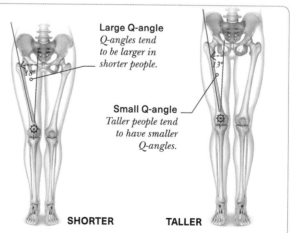

Large Q-angle
Q-angles tend to be larger in shorter people.

18°

Small Q-angle
Taller people tend to have smaller Q-angles.

13°

SHORTER　　**TALLER**

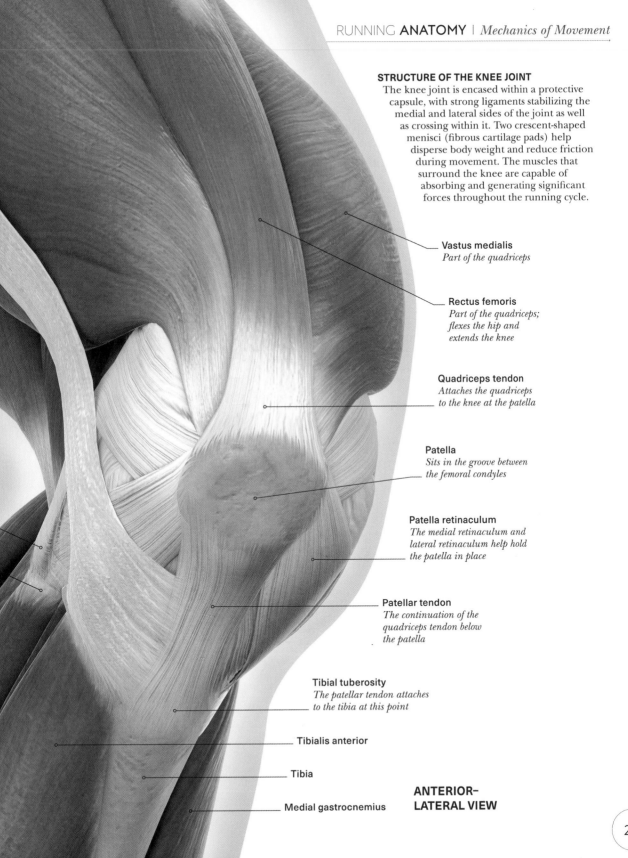

STRUCTURE OF THE KNEE JOINT

The knee joint is encased within a protective capsule, with strong ligaments stabilizing the medial and lateral sides of the joint as well as crossing within it. Two crescent-shaped menisci (fibrous cartilage pads) help disperse body weight and reduce friction during movement. The muscles that surround the knee are capable of absorbing and generating significant forces throughout the running cycle.

Vastus medialis
Part of the quadriceps

Rectus femoris
Part of the quadriceps; flexes the hip and extends the knee

Quadriceps tendon
Attaches the quadriceps to the knee at the patella

Patella
Sits in the groove between the femoral condyles

Patella retinaculum
The medial retinaculum and lateral retinaculum help hold the patella in place

Patellar tendon
The continuation of the quadriceps tendon below the patella

Tibial tuberosity
The patellar tendon attaches to the tibia at this point

Tibialis anterior

Tibia

Medial gastrocnemius

ANTERIOR–LATERAL VIEW

25

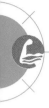

HIP

The head of the leg's femur bone fits into the pelvis at the hip, which is a synovial joint (see p.20). Although its ball-and-socket structure allows for a broad range of movement in all three planes, the hip joint's main function is to provide stability, as it must bear our body weight when we stand or move.

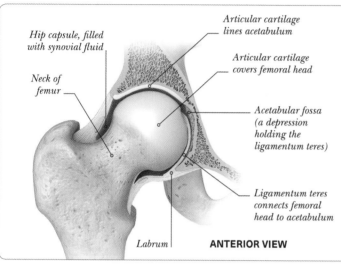

Hip capsule, filled with synovial fluid

Neck of femur

Articular cartilage lines acetabulum

Articular cartilage covers femoral head

Acetabular fossa (a depression holding the ligamentum teres)

Ligamentum teres connects femoral head to acetabulum

Labrum

ANTERIOR VIEW

Hip cross-section

The hip joint enables the swinging motion of the legs during running, as well as internal rotation during the early loading phase (see p.66). The deep acetabulum (the "socket") securely encompasses nearly the entire head of the femur (the "ball"), creating a large surface area within the joint, improving stability. The joint is surrounded by strong ligaments and a thick capsule of connective tissue. A horseshoe-shaped layer of fibrous cartilage (the labrum) borders the acetabulum, further increasing the depth of the socket.

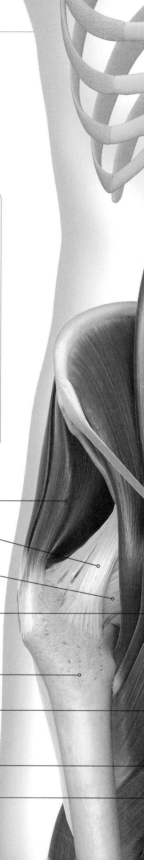

Gluteus minimus
The central layer of the three glutes; abducts the hip and stabilizes it

Iliofemoral ligament

Pubofemoral ligament

Pectineus
Attaches from pubic bone to femur; flexes and adducts the hip

Femur

Adductor longus
Attaches from the pubis to the back of the femur

Adductor magnus

**ANTERIOR VIEW
DEEP MUSCLES**

Gracilis

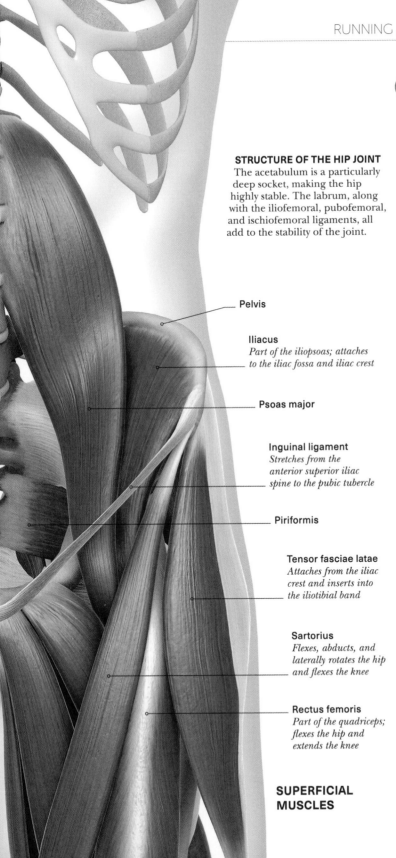

STRUCTURE OF THE HIP JOINT
The acetabulum is a particularly deep socket, making the hip highly stable. The labrum, along with the iliofemoral, pubofemoral, and ischiofemoral ligaments, all add to the stability of the joint.

Pelvis

Iliacus
Part of the iliopsoas; attaches to the iliac fossa and iliac crest

Psoas major

Inguinal ligament
Stretches from the anterior superior iliac spine to the pubic tubercle

Piriformis

Tensor fasciae latae
Attaches from the iliac crest and inserts into the iliotibial band

Sartorius
Flexes, abducts, and laterally rotates the hip and flexes the knee

Rectus femoris
Part of the quadriceps; flexes the hip and extends the knee

SUPERFICIAL MUSCLES

ANATOMICAL VARIATIONS
Hip socket impingement

The shape of the hip joint varies between individuals. The acetabulum can be deep or shallow; the femoral head can be round or cone-shaped. Some variations can lead to femoroacetabular impingement (FAI), in which the ball pinches against the socket at the anterior side of the joint, causing pain in the hip or groin area during certain complex movements in early loading (see p.66) involving a combination of flexion, adduction, and internal rotation.

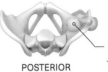

ANTERIOR

Hip socket and
femoral head

POSTERIOR
SUPERIOR VIEW

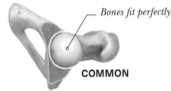

Bones fit perfectly

COMMON

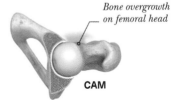

Bone overgrowth on femoral head

CAM

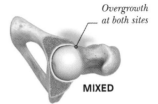

Overgrowth at both sites

MIXED

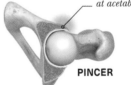

Bone overgrowth at acetabular rim

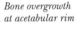

PINCER

PELVIS

The pelvis consists of two large, curved hip bones and the sacrum (tailbone), with three joints and a web of strong ligaments holding everything together in a bowl-like structure that protects the internal pelvic organs. Pelvic stability and alignment are important considerations for runners. The pelvis supports the weight of the upper body when you sit and transfers it to the legs when you stand. It also serves as an attachment point for many muscles in the trunk and legs.

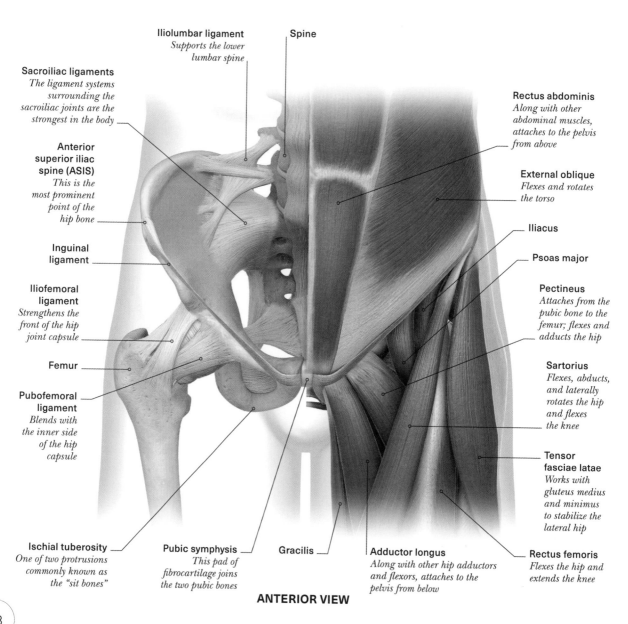

Iliolumbar ligament
Supports the lower lumbar spine

Spine

Sacroiliac ligaments
The ligament systems surrounding the sacroiliac joints are the strongest in the body

Rectus abdominis
Along with other abdominal muscles, attaches to the pelvis from above

Anterior superior iliac spine (ASIS)
This is the most prominent point of the hip bone

External oblique
Flexes and rotates the torso

Iliacus

Inguinal ligament

Psoas major

Iliofemoral ligament
Strengthens the front of the hip joint capsule

Pectineus
Attaches from the pubic bone to the femur; flexes and adducts the hip

Femur

Sartorius
Flexes, abducts, and laterally rotates the hip and flexes the knee

Pubofemoral ligament
Blends with the inner side of the hip capsule

Tensor fasciae latae
Works with gluteus medius and minimus to stabilize the lateral hip

Ischial tuberosity
One of two protrusions commonly known as the "sit bones"

Pubic symphysis
This pad of fibrocartilage joins the two pubic bones

Gracilis

Adductor longus
Along with other hip adductors and flexors, attaches to the pelvis from below

Rectus femoris
Flexes the hip and extends the knee

ANTERIOR VIEW

ANATOMICAL VARIATIONS

Position of sciatic nerve

There are various paths the sciatic nerve can take as it passes the piriformis muscle. It may pass below, above, or even through the piriformis and it may be divided or undivided. Some variations may contribute to entrapment of the sciatic nerve when the piriformis is tight due to prolonged running, producing pain deep in the buttock and posterior thigh (see Deep Gluteal Syndrome, p.62). The Modified Pigeon and Piriformis Ball Release stretches (see pp.90 and 94) can help bring relief.

Sciatic nerve passes beneath the piriformis

Divided nerve passes through and beneath

Divided nerve passes above and beneath piriformis

Complete nerve passes through

(A) COMMON   **(B)**   **(C)**   **(D)**

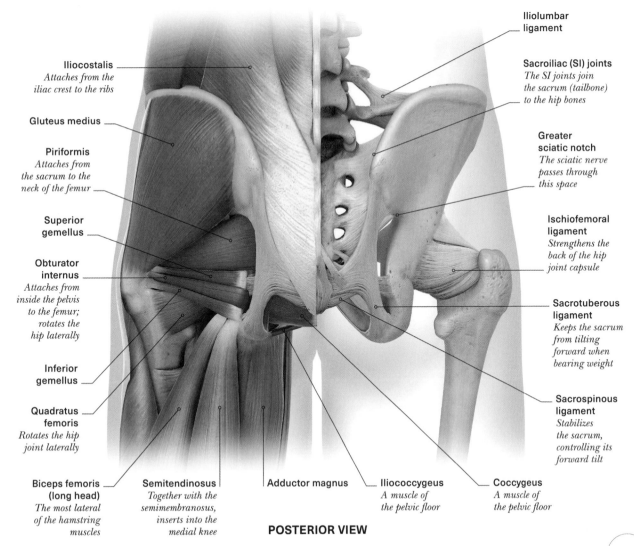

Iliolumbar ligament

Sacroiliac (SI) joints
The SI joints join the sacrum (tailbone) to the hip bones

Greater sciatic notch
The sciatic nerve passes through this space

Ischiofemoral ligament
Strengthens the back of the hip joint capsule

Sacrotuberous ligament
Keeps the sacrum from tilting forward when bearing weight

Sacrospinous ligament
Stabilizes the sacrum, controlling its forward tilt

Iliocostalis
Attaches from the iliac crest to the ribs

Gluteus medius

Piriformis
Attaches from the sacrum to the neck of the femur

Superior gemellus

Obturator internus
Attaches from inside the pelvis to the femur; rotates the hip laterally

Inferior gemellus

Quadratus femoris
Rotates the hip joint laterally

Biceps femoris (long head)
The most lateral of the hamstring muscles

Semitendinosus
Together with the semimembranosus, inserts into the medial knee

Adductor magnus

Iliococcygeus
A muscle of the pelvic floor

Coccygeus
A muscle of the pelvic floor

POSTERIOR VIEW

29

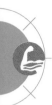

CORE

The muscles in the midsection of your body make up the core. This area coordinates the movements of upper and lower body. When you run, a well-functioning core allows you to control your trunk over your planted leg, maximizing the production, transfer, and control of force and motion to your lower limbs. The spine supports the trunk.

MUSCLES OF THE CORE
The core muscles are multilayered. The muscles that stabilize the trunk are situated deeply, whereas the muscles that create movement are closer to the surface.

Spine

The spine encases and protects the spinal cord and supports the body's weight. It is made up of three sections: cervical, thoracic, and lumbar. Its three natural curves combine to form an "S" shape, across which the body's weight is evenly distributed, enabling the spine to withstand stress. The different regions of the spine enable a range of movements involved in running (see p.147).

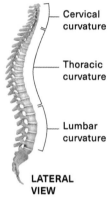

— Cervical curvature

— Thoracic curvature

— Lumbar curvature

LATERAL VIEW

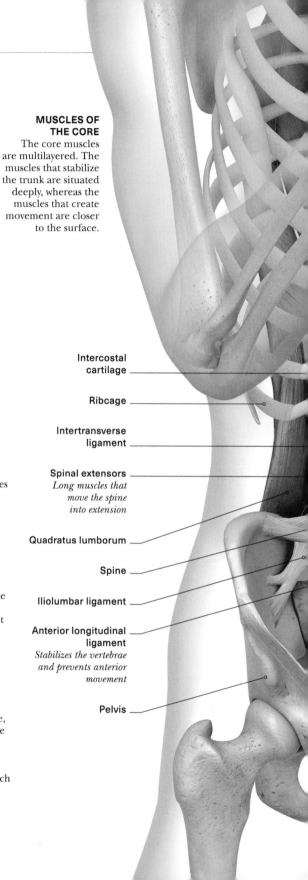

Intercostal cartilage

Ribcage

Intertransverse ligament

Spinal extensors
Long muscles that move the spine into extension

Quadratus lumborum

Spine

Iliolumbar ligament

Anterior longitudinal ligament
Stabilizes the vertebrae and prevents anterior movement

Pelvis

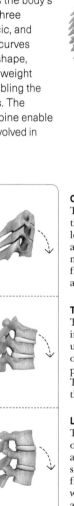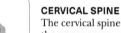

CERVICAL SPINE
The cervical spine comprises the upper seven vertebrae, located in the neck. These allow for a large range of movement: extension, flexion, side flexion, and rotation.

THORACIC SPINE
The central twelve vertebrae in the chest section make up the thoracic spine. Most of the torso's rotation is produced at these joints. The ribs attach to the thoracic spine.

LUMBAR SPINE
The lumbar spine consists of the five largest vertebrae, although some people have six. This section enables flexion and extension, as well as some side flexion and rotation, and bears much of the body's weight.

ANTERIOR VIEW   **LATERAL VIEW**

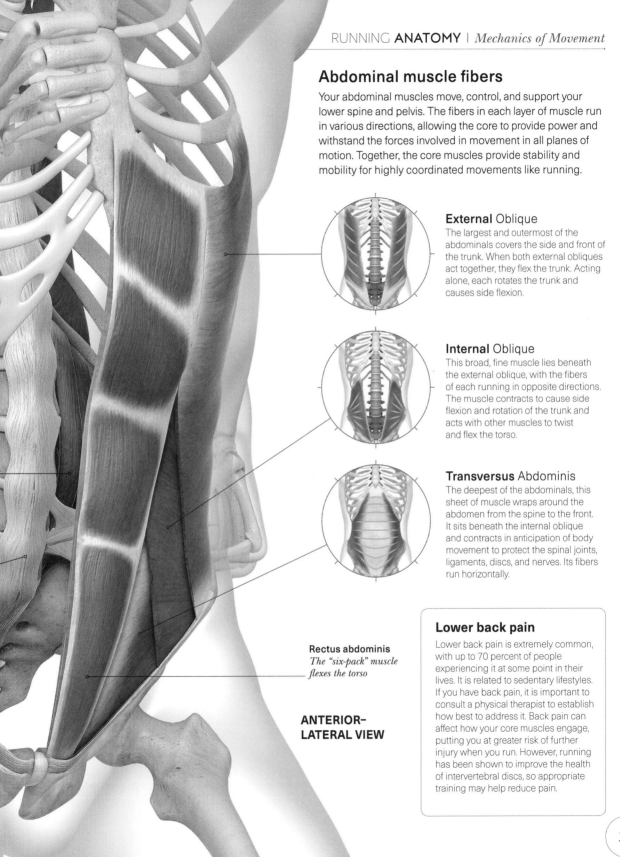

Abdominal muscle fibers

Your abdominal muscles move, control, and support your lower spine and pelvis. The fibers in each layer of muscle run in various directions, allowing the core to provide power and withstand the forces involved in movement in all planes of motion. Together, the core muscles provide stability and mobility for highly coordinated movements like running.

External Oblique

The largest and outermost of the abdominals covers the side and front of the trunk. When both external obliques act together, they flex the trunk. Acting alone, each rotates the trunk and causes side flexion.

Internal Oblique

This broad, fine muscle lies beneath the external oblique, with the fibers of each running in opposite directions. The muscle contracts to cause side flexion and rotation of the trunk and acts with other muscles to twist and flex the torso.

Transversus Abdominis

The deepest of the abdominals, this sheet of muscle wraps around the abdomen from the spine to the front. It sits beneath the internal oblique and contracts in anticipation of body movement to protect the spinal joints, ligaments, discs, and nerves. Its fibers run horizontally.

Rectus abdominis
The "six-pack" muscle flexes the torso

ANTERIOR–LATERAL VIEW

Lower back pain

Lower back pain is extremely common, with up to 70 percent of people experiencing it at some point in their lives. It is related to sedentary lifestyles. If you have back pain, it is important to consult a physical therapist to establish how best to address it. Back pain can affect how your core muscles engage, putting you at greater risk of further injury when you run. However, running has been shown to improve the health of intervertebral discs, so appropriate training may help reduce pain.

POWERING
MOVEMENT

Nutrients from the foods we eat, combined with oxygen from the air we breathe, provide the raw materials needed to generate the energy that powers movement. The body uses these resources in a complex interplay between the cardiorespiratory and digestive systems to deliver the muscles their power supply.

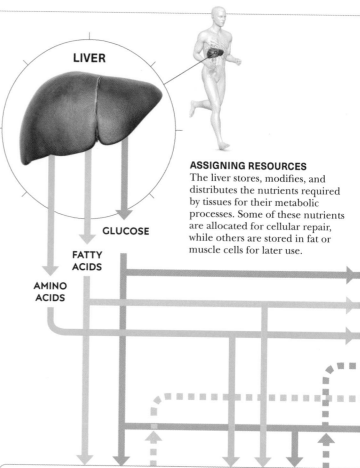

LIVER

GLUCOSE

FATTY ACIDS

AMINO ACIDS

ASSIGNING RESOURCES
The liver stores, modifies, and distributes the nutrients required by tissues for their metabolic processes. Some of these nutrients are allocated for cellular repair, while others are stored in fat or muscle cells for later use.

SOURCES
OF ENERGY

The stomach and intestines process the foods we consume. When running, we rely mostly on energy derived from carbohydrates, but in certain situations, the body uses fat and protein sources. Carbohydrates are processed and stored as glycogen in the liver and muscles. Fats are processed and stored in the liver as fatty acids (triglycerides) or as fat in adipose tissue. Proteins break down into amino acids and are the building blocks for new muscle tissue.

Increased glycogen stores

With proper training, the body learns to store higher levels of glycogen in the muscles and also becomes more efficient at conserving it at your race pace. This is particularly important when running for over 90 minutes, by which time glycogen stores are typically depleted. Because glycogen is the most efficient fuel source, it is advantageous to have it last for as long as possible.

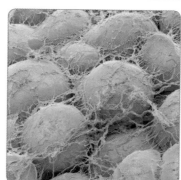

FAT CELLS
Energy-rich triglycerides are stored as fat in muscle and adipose tissue, then broken down into free fatty acids and released into the bloodstream when required, to be used by cells as an energy source. Excess glucose is also converted to fat.

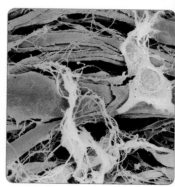

MUSCLE CELLS
Glycogen is stored in muscle cells, where it is later released to provide energy for muscle contractions. It is also released from muscle into the bloodstream to raise blood glucose levels if they fall.

LIVER PATHWAYS

▬▬ Glucose leaves
the liver to be used

■ ■ ■ Glucose released
from storage

▭▭ Fatty acids leave
the liver to be stored

▪ ▪ ▪ Fatty acids released
from storage

▬▬ Amino acids leave
the liver to be used

VER CELLS

:cess glucose is stored inside liver
lls as glycogen granules, which are
en released as required.

ACCESSING ENERGY

Muscle growth, renewal, and
repair, as well as contractions of
the major muscle groups when
running, all require energy.
The body draws a supply of the
appropriate energy directly from
the liver. However, if needed, a
back-up supply is available from
muscle and fat cells.

ENERGY SYSTEMS

The molecule adenosine triphosphate (ATP)
stores, transports, and releases the energy
used for muscle contractions. The body
has three ways of accessing ATP, or three
energy systems. The primary system it draws
on depends on the duration and intensity
of the exercise.

The first port of call is stored ATP in cells.
Muscle fibers store enough ATP to power
contractions for up to 10 seconds, providing
lots of energy rapidly, but for immediate,
short-term use and maximum intensity efforts
only. (Once used, it takes up to 5 minutes to
restore this supply.) When you start to run,
this system kicks in first to get you moving.

After the stored ATP is depleted, food
energy—usually glucose—is converted to
ATP within muscle cells and maintained in
steady supply, either through anaerobic or
aerobic cell respiration.

For high-intensity running, in which
the oxygen supply is unable to meet the
demand, the body uses anaerobic cell
respiration. This system fires up when you
start to run and powers movement until the
aerobic system (see below), which takes
longer to kick in, catches up.

Aerobic cell respiration is the primary
system used to power moderate- or low-
intensity work. It can draw on glucose stores
for up to 90 minutes. Distance running is
mostly an aerobic activity, but any time the
body needs a short burst of extra energy that
cannot be accommodated by the aerobic
system—when sprinting across the finish line
of a race, for instance—the body draws on
the anaerobic system.

Both aerobic and anaerobic respiration
begin with a process known as glycogenolysis,
which releases glucose from glycogen, after
which a chain reaction known as cell
respiration (see pp.34–35) takes place to
convert the glucose into ATP so that it is
available to power muscle contractions.

33

CELL RESPIRATION

Muscle cell respiration is so named because it takes place within muscle cells. First, glucose is released from glycogen, which has been stored within the muscle or supplied directly by the liver. The body then relies on either aerobic or anaerobic cell respiration to transform the glucose into the molecule ATP, which provides the energy needed for muscle contractions.

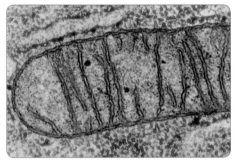

MITOCHONDRIA

Aerobic cell respiration takes place within mitochondria, making them the "workhorses" of the cell. These structures can increase in number and size with endurance training, improving the body's aerobic cell respiration efficiency.

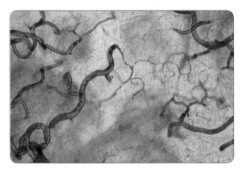

CAPILLARIES

Small branches of blood vessels, known as capillaries, deliver oxygen and nutrients to cells for aerobic respiration. Endurance training increases capillary density and function, which improves muscle endurance performance.

Aerobic and anaerobic respiration

In aerobic cell respiration, the body uses oxygen to convert glucose into ATP. During strenuous exercise, if there is a shortage of oxygen (due to inadequate delivery or high rate of use), the body relies on anaerobic respiration. While this process does not require oxygen, it does cause lactate accumulation. Far from being a metabolic waste product, lactate provides a valuable energy source when sufficient oxygen becomes available (once pace slows). Its accumulation causes a burning sensation in the muscles and induces fatigue, meaning anaerobic cell respiration is a limited resource.

ENDURANCE

AEROBIC RESPIRATION

Aerobic respiration has tremendous energy-yielding capacity and, as a result, is the primary method of energy production during endurance exercise. A total of approximately 38 ATP molecules can be generated from one molecule of glycogen.

2 ATP molecules

The first stage of aerobic cell respiration takes place in the cytoplasm within the cells of muscles. This process of glycolysis breaks down glucose into pyruvic acid, generating 2 ATP molecules for use. The pyruvic acid then moves into the cell's mitochondria for the next stage of aerobic cell respiration.

OXYGEN →

FATTY ACIDS →

AMINO ACIDS →

→ *AEROBIC RESPIRATION IN MITOCHONDRIA*

36 ATP molecules

In order to process the pyruvic acid, a series of chemical reactions takes place within the cell's mitochondria in the presence of oxygen, which generates 36 ATP molecules. Water and carbon dioxide are also generated as byproducts and are cleared by the body.

ENDURANCE

 Lactate threshold

During steady-state exercise, aerobic cell respiration matches the energy needs of muscles. When intensity increases beyond the capacity of aerobic respiration, blood lactate accumulation begins to rise exponentially. Your lactate threshold (LT) represents the highest intensity you can manage before your body begins to exponentially accumulate lactate. Your LT significantly contributes to your distance-running capacity because it reflects the rate at which your muscles can sustain aerobic energy production.

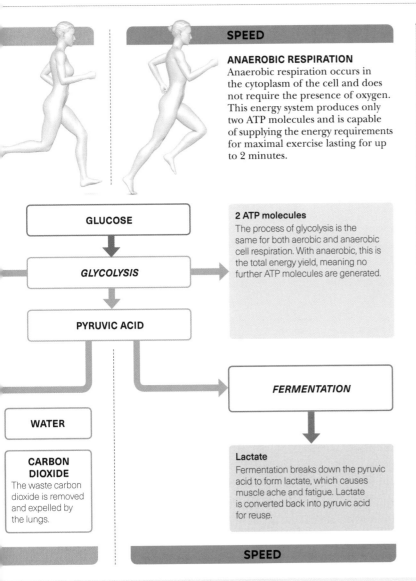

SPEED

ANAEROBIC RESPIRATION
Anaerobic respiration occurs in the cytoplasm of the cell and does not require the presence of oxygen. This energy system produces only two ATP molecules and is capable of supplying the energy requirements for maximal exercise lasting for up to 2 minutes.

| GLUCOSE |
| *GLYCOLYSIS* |
| PYRUVIC ACID |

WATER

CARBON DIOXIDE
The waste carbon dioxide is removed and expelled by the lungs.

2 ATP molecules
The process of glycolysis is the same for both aerobic and anaerobic cell respiration. With anaerobic, this is the total energy yield, meaning no further ATP molecules are generated.

FERMENTATION

Lactate
Fermentation breaks down the pyruvic acid to form lactate, which causes muscle ache and fatigue. Lactate is converted back into pyruvic acid for reuse.

SPEED

Metabolizing fats
When glycogen stores run out, muscle cells turn to fat for energy. The body's fat stores can deliver up to 30 times more energy than its glycogen reserves. To be used for energy, triglycerides must be broken down into free fatty acids in a process called lypolysis, then circulated in the bloodstream to reach the muscles for cell respiration.

Efficient use of fat stores
Endurance training increases the body's metabolism of fat for energy during both rest and submaximal (steady-state aerobic) exercise. In endurance runners, this adaptation enables the body to conserve the glycogen stores that are important during prolonged runs. The body can store only a limited quantity of glycogen, so it is an advantage to be able to metabolize fats efficiently during prolonged submaximal exercise.

"Hitting the wall" is the feeling of sudden and dramatic fatigue when the body runs out of glycogen. Enhancing the body's ability to utilize fat stores allows it to preserve glycogen stores and so delay hitting the wall—or avoid it altogether.

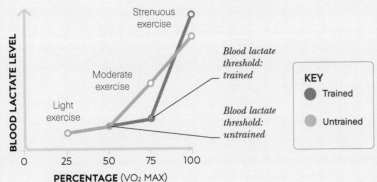

PERCENTAGE (VO₂ MAX)

BLOOD LACTATE CONCENTRATION
This chart shows blood lactate levels in trained and untrained subjects at varying exercise intensities, expressed as a percentage of maximal oxygen consumption (VO₂ max, see p.37). Regular training shifts the blood lactate accumulation curve to the right. Trained muscle can withstand higher levels of intensity before blood lactate accumulation occurs. Recognizing your LT by pace or feel (see pp.164–166) allows you to avoid the exponential increase in blood lactate and associated fatigue.

OXYGEN DELIVERY

Major organ systems work as a unit to supply the oxygen needed to power muscle contractions. Oxygen enters the bloodstream via the lungs and is delivered to working muscles. Here, it is exchanged for carbon dioxide, which is carried back to the lungs to be exhaled. The pumping action of the heart maintains this vital circulation of blood.

HEAD AND UPPER BODY

Veins
Return deoxygenated blood from the head and upper body to the heart

Arteries
Deliver oxygenated blood to the upper body

RIGHT LUNG

LEFT LUNG

HEART

Pulmonary artery
Delivers deoxygenated blood to the lungs for expulsion of carbon dioxide

Pulmonary vein
Carries oxygenated blood from the lungs to the heart for circulation

LIVER

Arteries
Deliver oxygenated blood to the lower body

HEART AND CIRCULATION
Arteries (shown in red) carry oxygenated blood away from the heart, while veins (shown in blue) carry deoxygenated blood toward the heart. This is reversed in the pulmonary loop of the circulatory system, which connects the heart and lungs.

GASTRO-INTESTINAL TRACT

Capillaries
Oxygen diffuses into tissues in exchange for carbon dioxide

Artery wall
Thick muscular wall changes diameter to regulate blood flow

Veins
Return deoxygenated blood from the legs to the heart

LOWER BODY

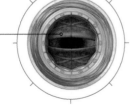

Vein valve
One-way valves prevent backflow

Vein
Veins carry deoxygenated blood from working muscles to the heart and lungs for the removal of carbon dioxide and heat.

Capillary
Capillary networks connect arteries and veins with tissue cells. This is where the exchange of oxygen for waste products takes place.

Artery
Arteries carry oxygen-rich blood from the heart and lungs to working muscles.

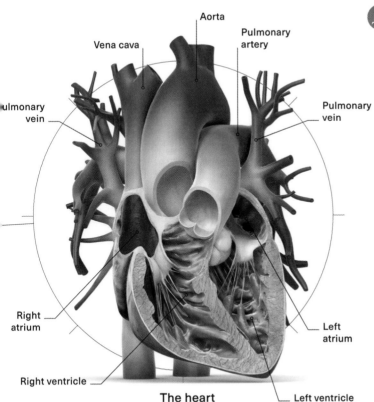

Aorta

Vena cava

Pulmonary artery

Pulmonary vein

Pulmonary vein

Right atrium

Left atrium

Right ventricle

Left ventricle
Pumps oxygenated blood around the body

The heart

The heart maintains the rate of blood circulation to match the body's varying demand for oxygen. During exercise, the rate and strength of cardiac muscle contractions increases to maximize blood circulation, allowing for greater oxygen consumption. Training increases the size of the left ventricle to enable the heart to accommodate greater blood volumes.

VO₂ max

Your VO₂ max is a measure of how much oxygen your body can consume during maximal effort. A high VO₂ max score means the quantity of oxygen available in the muscles for aerobic cell respiration is comparatively large. The body's ability to transport oxygen to muscles depends on four factors: maximum heart rate, stroke volume (the amount of blood pumped from the heart with one heartbeat), quantity of hemoglobin (which carries oxygen) in the blood, and the proportion of the circulation that is transported to your working muscles. Some of these factors can be improved with training, while others are genetically determined.

Training adaptations

Training causes physical adaptations that result in improvements in the energy systems that power movement.

Aerobic training

The aim of aerobic training (see pp.180–182, 186–187) is to increase the body's efficiency at aerobic cell respiration, enabling you to maintain this system for longer during exercise before anaerobic cell respiration kicks in. This improves aerobic endurance and VO₂ max. Adaptations result in:

- Lactate accumulation occurring at higher exercise intensities
- More rapid rate of lactate clearance
- Increased stroke volume
- Increased blood volume
- Increased red blood cell volume, enhancing oxygen delivery
- Increased capillarization of muscles (see p.34)
- Increased mitochondria (see p.34) in number and size, allowing for improved aerobic cell respiration
- Increased oxidative enzyme activity of mitochondria, improving the efficiency of mitochondria
- Increased efficiency of existing capillaries
- Improved blood redistribution
- Increased size of slow-twitch muscle fibers (see p.19)
- Increased myoglobin content of muscle (allowing increased oxygen levels to muscles)

Anaerobic training

Anaerobic training (see pp.183–185) increases your body's ability to tolerate and clear blood lactate and also increases your lactate threshold (see pp.34–35). Adaptations result in:

- Increased muscular strength
- Improved mechanical efficiency
- Increased muscle oxidative capacity
- Increased muscle buffering capacity (enabling muscles to withstand the build-up of acidity that occurs as part of the cellular respiration process)
- Increased lactate clearance capacity

CONTROLLING
MOVEMENT

The brain and nervous system work together with the endocrine system to enable and coordinate both consciously and unconsciously controlled movements during running. They also play an important role in maintaining a state of equilibrium within the body.

THE **CONTROL NETWORK**

The brain is the body's control center. It sends and receives messages via the spinal cord and peripheral nervous system (PNS). The PNS has two divisions: the autonomic nervous system (ANS) and the somatic nervous system. The somatic nervous system includes both motor and sensory fibers to control voluntary movement of skeletal muscle. The ANS controls involuntary processes such as temperature regulation, breathing, and the regulation of heart rate.

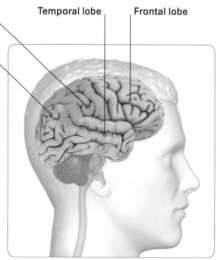

Brain
Controls movement

Thyroid
Regulates metabolism

Parathyroid
Regulates blood calcium

Heart
Pumps blood to the body

Adrenal glands
Regulate metabolism and immune system and produce adrenaline

Pancreas
Regulates blood sugar

Small intestine
Absorbs nutrients from food

Gonads
Produce sex hormones

Peripheral nerves
Motor and sensory nerves form a network throughout the body

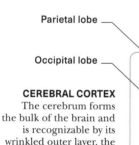

Parietal lobe

Temporal lobe

Frontal lobe

Occipital lobe

CEREBRAL CORTEX
The cerebrum forms the bulk of the brain and is recognizable by its wrinkled outer layer, the cerebral cortex. Areas responsible for motor and sensory control are located in the frontal and parietal lobes respectively.
When you run, your motor cortex works with the spinal cord and other brain regions to control movement.

NEURO-ENDOCRINE SYSTEM
Peripheral nerves carry information from all parts of the body to the brain for processing, as well as instructions to the body to control movement. The brain also works with the endocrine system to manage internal conditions in response to changes within the body to retain internal balance.

Pineal gland
*Helps regulate
circadian rhythm*

Hypothalamus
*Regulates body
temperature*

Cerebellum
*Coordinates and
regulates motor actions*

Pituitary gland
*Controls the action
of other glands*

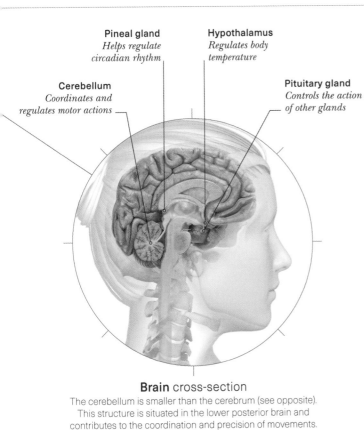

Brain cross-section
The cerebellum is smaller than the cerebrum (see opposite).
This structure is situated in the lower posterior brain and
contributes to the coordination and precision of movements.
Important glands are also situated in the brain.

HOW WE MOVE

The motor cortex (located at the
rear of the frontal lobe) coordinates
muscle activity for both involuntary
and voluntary movement. Signals sent
via motor neurons in the spinal cord
and peripheral nerves tell muscles to
contract and relax as necessary. When
you run, your motor cortex controls a
finely coordinated and rapid sequence
of motor-neuron firings, which cause
specific muscles to contract in order
to create the required movements.

*Muscle fibers
running in
parallel*

*Motor neuron
stimulates the
muscle to contract*

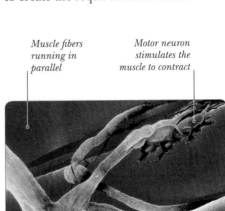

NEUROMUSCULAR JUNCTION
Each motor neuron meets with the muscle
fiber it innervates at a neuromuscular junction,
where it transmits the nerve impulses that initiate
muscle contractions. Skeletal muscle fibers
usually each possess one neuromuscular junction.

Spinal cord
*The body's main
communication
pathway*

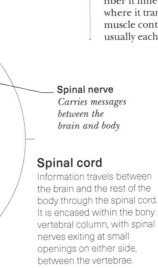

Spinal nerve
*Carries messages
between the
brain and body*

Spinal cord
Information travels between
the brain and the rest of the
body through the spinal cord.
It is encased within the bony
vertebral column, with spinal
nerves exiting at small
openings on either side,
between the vertebrae.

Vertebra
*Encases the
spinal cord to
protect it*

BALANCE AND COORDINATION

How we balance and synchronize movements relies on the integration of sensory and motor information, often at the subconscious level. For instance, as your weight shifts during running, structures in your inner ear, in combination with visual input, coordinate with your brain in order to maintain balance. Meanwhile, motor input to your legs adjusts the stiffness of your lower limbs to accommodate changes in the terrain. These constant adjustments allow you to maintain a level head and prioritize vision.

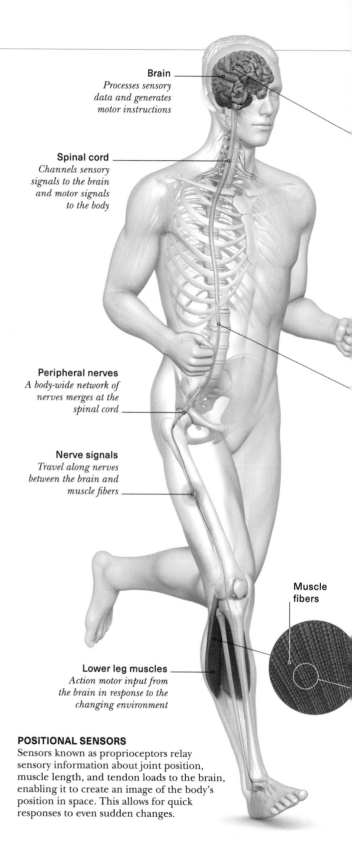

Brain
Processes sensory data and generates motor instructions

Spinal cord
Channels sensory signals to the brain and motor signals to the body

Peripheral nerves
A body-wide network of nerves merges at the spinal cord

Nerve signals
Travel along nerves between the brain and muscle fibers

Muscle fibers

Lower leg muscles
Action motor input from the brain in response to the changing environment

Evolved to run

There is evidence in the human anatomy to support the idea that we evolved the capacity to run long distances. Examples include the optimization of energy use, stabilization of the trunk and head, and regulation of body temperature. The nuchal ligament is one structural modification that was absent in our ape ancestors; another is our comparatively long Achilles tendon.

Nuchal ligament
This structure evolved to prevent the head from tipping forward during activities such as running

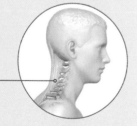

Achilles tendon
The Achilles' energy storage and return properties may have evolved in response to endurance running

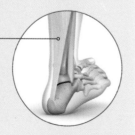

POSITIONAL SENSORS

Sensors known as proprioceptors relay sensory information about joint position, muscle length, and tendon loads to the brain, enabling it to create an image of the body's position in space. This allows for quick responses to even sudden changes.

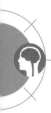

Sensory cortex
Receives and processes sensory information relating to touch, pain, and temperature

Motor cortex
Generates instructions for voluntary movement

Motor and sensory cortices

Located in the cerebral cortex (see p.38), the motor cortex is involved in planning, coordinating, and controlling voluntary motion. It sits beside the sensory cortex, which processes and integrates sensory data from the body.

MIDCORONAL VIEW

Motor neuron
Relays nerve signals to muscle fibers

Interneurons
Connect nerves to the spinal cord

Sensory neuron
Carries impulses from peripheral nerves

Spinal cord

There are three main types of nerve cells in the spinal cord. Sensory neurons pass sensory data from the body to the brain. Motor neurons carry instructions from the brain to skeletal muscle fibers to control movement. Both communicate with the central nervous system (CNS) via interneurons.

Motor signals from the brain

Sensory signals to the brain

Muscle spindle fiber
Detects changes in the muscle's length

Sensory neuron
Relays sensory information to the brain

Muscle cell

Muscle spindles

These receptors within muscles pick up information about changes in muscle length and tension to relay to the CNS. Through a reflex action, they also prevent muscles from overstretching by initiating a stronger counter-contraction.

Balance

Loop-shaped, fluid-filled canals in the inner ear contain hairlike sensors that detect movement in three planes. The signals they send to the brain enable it to monitor the position of the head in space as you move. They also detect sudden deviations, such as when you step off a curb while running. The brain interprets this information in conjunction with other sensory data and coordinates the appropriate response to retain balance and keep the head level.

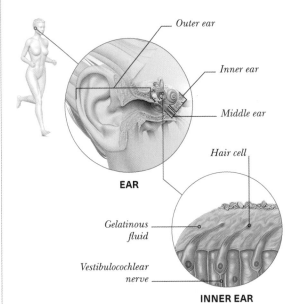

Outer ear

Inner ear

Middle ear

EAR

Hair cell

Gelatinous fluid

Vestibulocochlear nerve

INNER EAR

DIRECTION OF MOVEMENT
Gelatinous fluid surrounds tiny hairlike sensors within the otolithic membrane of the inner ear. As the head moves, the movement of the fluid around the sensors enables them to pick up information that allows the brain to determine the direction of the movement.

Vision and coordination

Your eyes work in the same way as other sensors do, passing sensory input (in this case, visual) to the brain for processing. This allows you to anticipate the terrain ahead and plan for changes in it or to navigate around moving objects such as dogs or crowds. Much of this coordination happens at the subconscious level. Maintaining a level head, despite the impact from each step, accommodates this function.

UNCONSCIOUS FUNCTIONS

As well as conscious movement, the brain and nervous system also control the many unconscious functions that support exercise. The autonomic nervous system (ANS) regulates body temperature, breathing, and heart rate in the background while we run. It is divided into the sympathetic and parasympathetic nervous systems. During exercise, the sympathetic nervous system is mainly active, accelerating heart rate, dilating blood vessels and airways, and inhibiting digestion.

Homeostasis

Homeostasis is the state of internal equilibrium that the body works to retain despite changing conditions. The ANS coordinates with the endocrine system to release hormones into the bloodstream to maintain homeostasis. Hormones are chemical messengers that influence cellular functions. They control a number of physiological reactions in the body, including energy metabolism and tissue growth.

Hormonal balance

The endocrine system regulates hormone production so that they are available as required to carry out their vital functions. Overtraining can disrupt hormonal balance. Proper training requires a balance between overload and recovery (see p.169). If there is too much overload or not enough recovery, physical and psychological symptoms can result, manifesting as overtraining syndrome, a disorder that disrupts both the nervous system and hormones.

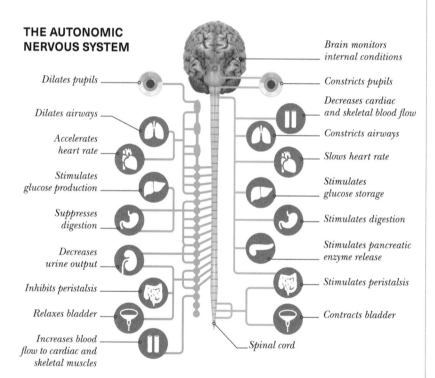

THE AUTONOMIC NERVOUS SYSTEM

Dilates pupils

Dilates airways

Accelerates heart rate

Stimulates glucose production

Suppresses digestion

Decreases urine output

Inhibits peristalsis

Relaxes bladder

Increases blood flow to cardiac and skeletal muscles

Brain monitors internal conditions

Constricts pupils

Decreases cardiac and skeletal blood flow

Constricts airways

Slows heart rate

Stimulates glucose storage

Stimulates digestion

Stimulates pancreatic enzyme release

Stimulates peristalsis

Contracts bladder

Spinal cord

SYMPATHETIC NERVOUS SYSTEM
Known for the "fight-or-flight" response it initiates, this system sustains functions during stress. Heart rate and strength of contractions increase, airways and blood vessels to the heart and muscles dilate, and glucose is released into the bloodstream to boost muscle power.

PARASYMPATHETIC NERVOUS SYSTEM
This is the body's ongoing maintenance system and plays a role in recovery after exercise. It contributes to processes such as digestion, urination, and energy conservation. Its effects tend to oppose those of the sympathetic nervous system.

> ### Supplementing hormones
>
> Although supplementation is often associated with doping in sports, there are situations in which a physician would advise you to supplement your own hormone production for health reasons.
>
> **Estrogen**
> Overtraining can reduce estrogen levels in women. In female runners suffering from RED-S (see p.63), estrogen levels drop dramatically, resulting in loss of bone mass and increased risk of musculoskeletal injury. It can be supplemented with a patch or the birth control pill to normalize estrogen levels and reduce injury risk.
>
> **Thyroxine**
> Both the condition of hypothyroidism and overtraining can reduce circulating levels of thyroxine, resulting in reduced metabolic rate and protein synthesis. Thyroid hormone replacement is usually prescribed to promote balance.
>
> **Insulin**
> Insulin regulates the entry of glucose into the body's tissues. Without it, only trace amounts of glucose enter cells, with catastrophic results. Diabetes affects the production and/ or function of insulin. Supplementing insulin is a common treatment.

Hormones that affect training

HORMONE	PRODUCTION SITE	FUNCTION
CORTISOL	adrenal glands	• Stimulates the production of glucose, at the expense of proteins and lipids If you overtrain, too much cortisol floods the body, leading to excessive protein breakdown and sleep problems and, potentially, increased feelings of stress.
TESTOSTERONE	mainly the testes in men and the adrenal glands and ovaries in women	• Increases muscle mass and bone mass • In elevated levels, creates larger muscle fibers and decreases recovery time from workouts If you train too hard, the pituitary gland turns off production until you have recovered. Present in higher levels in men than in women.
ESTROGEN	mainly the ovaries in women and the adrenal glands and testes in men	• Facilitates the breakdown of stored fat into fuel • Helps maintain bone density Present in higher levels in women than men.
ERYTHROPOIETIN	kidney	• Stimulates bone marrow to produce red blood cells, which carry oxygen from the lungs to the muscle cells, thereby increasing oxygen-carrying capacity
ENDORPHINS	pituitary gland and CNS	• Produces "runner's high" (see p.213), a feeling of euphoria associated with prolonged endurance training The body adapts to endorphins, so over time, we produce less with the same level of stimulation.
ADRENALINE (ALSO KNOWN AS EPINEPHRINE)	adrenal glands	• Triggers fight-or-flight response: increases heart rate, relaxes airways, contracts blood vessels, and stimulates the breakdown of muscle glycogen and fat—functions that are useful to competition runners
THYROXINE	thyroid gland	• Plays a major role in determining metabolic rate and maintaining muscle, brain, and overall hormonal function Thyroxine balance must be maintained to ensure muscles contract normally.
INSULIN	pancreas	• Causes cells to take up glucose from the bloodstream and either use it as fuel or store it as glycogen in muscles and liver
ATRIAL NATRIURETIC PEPTIDE	cardiac muscle	• Helps regulate blood pressure When you are running, your systolic blood pressure increases, as there is a greater demand on your heart to pump oxygenated blood around your body for bodily function, especially for muscle metabolism.
GROWTH HORMONE	pituitary gland	• Affects protein synthesis, muscle mass, bone density, tendon and ligament strength, and other functions vital for running The body adapts to GH, so the more you train, the less your body will produce GH at the same level, meaning you'll have to work harder to release the same quantities.

TEMPERATURE **CONTROL**

Humans are homeothermic, meaning that our internal body temperature must be maintained within a narrow range for survival. This can be challenging when faced with extreme temperatures. During exercise, heat is generated and must be eliminated from the body to maintain core temperature within reasonable limits. If this is not done adequately, the result may be some form of heat illness or possibly even death. At the very least, performance will be affected. If environmental conditions are at the extreme of temperature, relative humidity, or both, thermoregulation is much harder to accomplish.

THERMOREGULATION

Sensory receptors detect when the body's internal temperature deviates from its optimum level. In response, the hypothalamus sets off the appropriate corrective response in order to return the body to homeostasis. As internal conditions normalize, the hypothalamus deactivates the corrective measures.

Body increases internal temperature

The hypothalamus stimulates heat-generating processes in order to increase internal temperature:

- **Blood vessels at the surface constrict** (vasoconstriction), narrowing in order to minimize blood flow to the skin and restrict the transference of heat from the blood to the atmosphere by radiation.
- **Muscles produce shivering**, which generates heat.
- **Metabolism increases** in response to hormonal stimulation to increase heat generation.

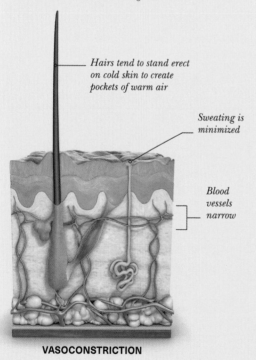

Hairs tend to stand erect on cold skin to create pockets of warm air

Sweating is minimized

Blood vessels narrow

VASOCONSTRICTION

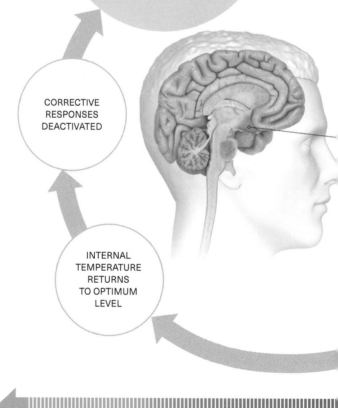

INTERNAL TEMPERATURE CHANGES

When you run, the activity raises internal temperature. If running in cold conditions, body temperature may reduce if you are inadequately protected from the cold. Internal body temperature must be maintained between 98°F (37°C) and 100°F (37.8°C).

CORRECTIVE RESPONSES DEACTIVATED

INTERNAL TEMPERATURE RETURNS TO OPTIMUM LEVEL

INTERNAL TEMPERATURE TOO LOW

Heat exposure

Exposure to the combination of environmental heat stress and internal heat generation can lead to either heat exhaustion or heatstroke. Symptoms of heat exhaustion include fatigue, dizziness, nausea, and a weak, rapid pulse. The thermoregulatory functions still function in heat exhaustion but cannot dissipate heat quickly enough. Heatstroke is a life-threatening illness that requires immediate medical management. It is caused by a failure of the body's thermoregulatory mechanisms and is characterized by cessation of sweating, as well as a rapid pulse and respiration rate, and accompanied by confusion, disorientation, or loss of consciousness.

Training adaptations

With specific training, the body's tolerance to exercising in hot conditions improves. The sensitivity of the sweat rate/core temperature relationship increases so that sweating occurs at lower core temperatures, keeping core temperature well within controllable levels. If you plan to race in a climate that is hotter than the one you are accustomed to training in, consider a heat acclimation protocol—such as using a hot tub or sauna after training or training in a heat chamber—to help improve your performance in the racing climate.

RECEPTORS
DETECT
THE CHANGE

**INTERNAL
TEMPERATURE
REGULATION**

HYPOTHALAMUS

This important endocrine gland is situated in the brain and is the body's thermoregulatory center. It stimulates the appropriate response in order to return the body's internal temperature to normal.

CORRECTIVE
RESPONSES
ACTIVATED

When the hypothalamus is unable to set off the appropriate corrective responses, core temperature continues to rise or fall beyond the desired window.

INTERNAL TEMPERATURE
TOO HIGH

Body decreases internal temperature

The hypothalamus stimulates heat-loss processes in order to decrease internal temperature:

- **Sweating increases** so the body can cool down as the moisture evaporates. Sweating is the body's primary method of dissipating the heat produced from strenuous exercise. Dehydration may impair the body's capacity to sweat and lose body heat. Hot, humid environments or inappropriate clothing may compromise the ability to lose heat from the body.

- **Blood vessels at the surface dilate** (vasodilation), widening to increase blood flow to the skin, from where heat can be transferred to the atmosphere by radiation. Increased blood flow to the skin shunts blood flow away from working muscles. This means there is less oxygen-rich blood available for powering movement.

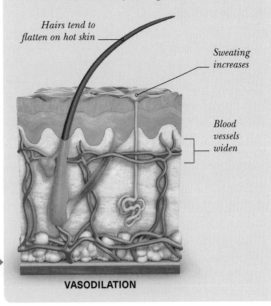

Hairs tend to flatten on hot skin

Sweating increases

Blood vessels widen

VASODILATION

EXTERNAL FACTORS

Various external factors affect runners. Impact forces act on the body each time the foot hits the ground. These must be countered by muscle contractions (see pp.18–19) and variations in our biomechanics. Also, the environment through which we run—its weather, terrain, and altitude—determines the work our bodies must do.

GROUND REACTION FORCE

Running involves a cyclical series of impacts. Once gravity pulls us to earth, we apply a force on the ground that is met with an equal and opposite ground reaction force (GRF). This force is applied to the body in a direction that consists of vertical, anterior-posterior (or propulsion-braking), and mediolateral (or side-to-side) components. Many injuries have been attributed to the GRF—to both its magnitude and the rate of its application—as the body must absorb this force while storing and transferring as much of its energy as possible into pushing back off the ground. Some studies have linked the vertical GRF loading rate with injury, while others have found associations between injury and the braking (posterior) force.

GRF distribution

The GRF is absorbed mostly within the lower limbs, although its effects extend through the entire body. How the body lands affects the way in which the GRF is distributed through the body. The posture of the lower limbs during the loading phase of the running cycle (see p.66) determines where the forces are directed. Where these forces are felt affects how our lower limbs move in order to absorb that load. For instance, longer step lengths produce greater braking forces. Landing with more knee flexion requires more strength in the quadriceps but reduces the forces felt above the knee.

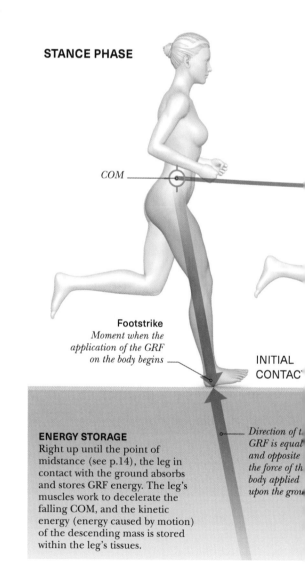

STANCE PHASE

COM

Footstrike
Moment when the application of the GRF on the body begins

INITIAL CONTAC

ENERGY STORAGE
Right up until the point of midstance (see p.14), the leg in contact with the ground absorbs and stores GRF energy. The leg's muscles work to decelerate the falling COM, and the kinetic energy (energy caused by motion) of the descending mass is stored within the leg's tissues.

Direction of t. GRF is equal and opposite the force of th body applied upon the grou

Storing and transferring energy

With each footstrike, the leg absorbs the GRF energy, then uses it to propel the body into the air. During the first half of stance phase, the body's center of mass (COM) descends. The joints flex while the viscoelastic tissues within the leg, such as the Achilles tendon, stretch under the weight of the descending body mass as they store the GRF energy (see p.18). The COM is at its lowest point at midstance. During the second half of stance phase, the stored energy is released (see p.19) to accelerate the COM into the air against gravity.

Minimizing forces

Despite numerous studies, researchers have been unable to determine an optimal gait pattern for reducing the injury risk associated with the GRF. That being said, a rear-foot strike pattern (see p.72), increased vertical oscillation (see p.71), and a longer step length (see p.70) have all been linked to higher rates of vertical GRF. Longer step lengths and forefoot striking (see p.72) have been associated with increased braking forces. One intervention that seems to reduce both vertical and braking forces is to increase your cadence (see p.70).

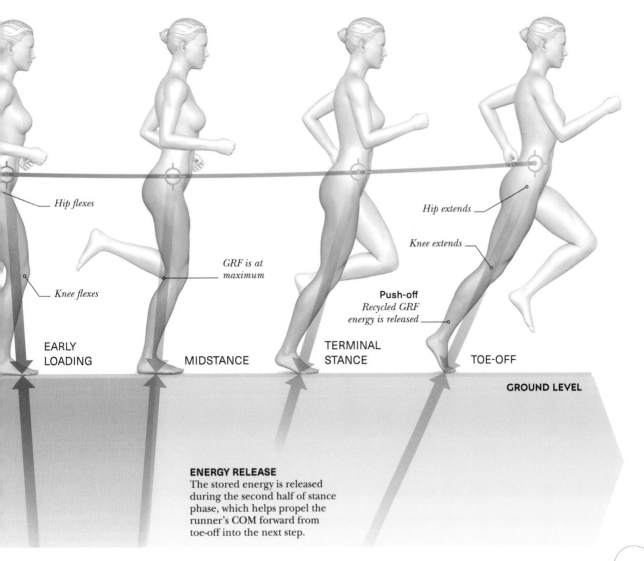

Hip flexes

Knee flexes

GRF is at maximum

Push-off
Recycled GRF energy is released

Hip extends

Knee extends

EARLY LOADING

MIDSTANCE

TERMINAL STANCE

TOE-OFF

GROUND LEVEL

ENERGY RELEASE
The stored energy is released during the second half of stance phase, which helps propel the runner's COM forward from toe-off into the next step.

Torque

When the GRF is applied to the body, it causes rotational forces ("torques" or "moments") to act on joints. Torque is a measure of how much a force acting on an object causes that object to rotate about an axis (the pivot point). The force might be applied at any distance from this pivot point, and its magnitude and direction cause the object (the lever arm) to rotate around the axis accordingly. This "external moment" must be countered by an "internal moment" applied to the lever. When running, the ankle and knee are pivot points and the feet and lower legs are levers. Where the GRF passes relative to the pivot point determines the direction of the external moment applied to the lever. The muscles around the pivotal joint must generate the power (the internal moment) needed to resist this movement. The interplay between these forces determines the lever's direction of movement.

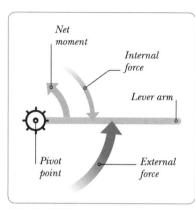

NET MOMENTS

In this example, the external moment (from the GRF) is greater than the internal counter moment (muscle action). The interplay between these two forces results in the net moment, which is the amount and direction of rotation of the lever arm (lower leg or foot) around the pivot point (knee or ankle joint).

KEY
◄ Internal moment
◄ External moment
◄ Ground reaction force
◄ Net moment

Knee

At initial contact, the GRF travels in a direction that passes behind the knee. This force on the lower leg encourages the knee to flex. In response, the quadriceps work eccentrically (see p.18) to generate a knee extension moment to control the rate of flexion. Eccentric strength training exercises focused on the quads build capacity for this response.

Rear-foot strike

When you land on your heel, the GRF travels behind the ankle joint, encouraging the ankle to plantarflex (see p.72). In response, the tibialis anterior works eccentrically (see p.18) to generate an ankle dorsiflexion moment to control the rate of plantarflexion.

REAR-FOOT STRIKE

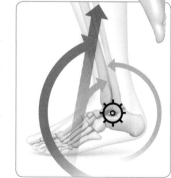

Forefoot strike

When you land on your forefoot, the GRF travels in front of the ankle joint, encouraging the ankle to dorsiflex (see p.72). In response, the calf muscles work eccentrically (see p.18) to generate an ankle plantarflexion moment to control the rate of dorsiflexion.

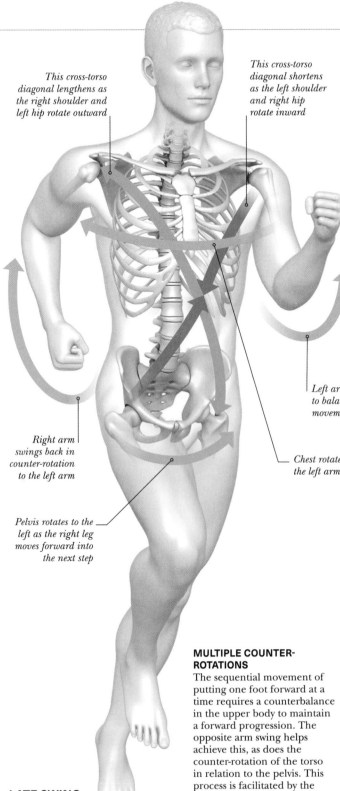

This cross-torso diagonal lengthens as the right shoulder and left hip rotate outward

This cross-torso diagonal shortens as the left shoulder and right hip rotate inward

Left arm drives forward to balance the forward movement of the right leg

Right arm swings back in counter-rotation to the left arm

Chest rotates to the right as the left arm drives through

Pelvis rotates to the left as the right leg moves forward into the next step

Diagonal elastic support

As rotational forces travel across the body during running, the body's counter-rotation causes the torso to stretch diagonally, and alternate this diagonal stretch with each stride. These movements transfer forces from the lower limbs to the upper limbs and back again. The layered alignment of muscles in the torso enables them to both produce and absorb the force of these rotations. The diagonal muscle-fiber orientation of the internal and external obliques and the latissimus dorsi and thoracolumbar fascia in the back also contribute. The winding up of the torso in one direction helps supply the energy for the unwinding in the opposite direction.

MULTIPLE COUNTER-ROTATIONS

The sequential movement of putting one foot forward at a time requires a counterbalance in the upper body to maintain a forward progression. The opposite arm swing helps achieve this, as does the counter-rotation of the torso in relation to the pelvis. This process is facilitated by the diagonal support mechanism.

LATE SWING

Rotation through kinetic chain

The kinetic chain is a concept that describes the body as a chain of linked segments. Each segment makes a small individual movement, and these link up with adjoining segments into larger movements along the chain. As you run, your body responds to the GRF and rotational forces acting on it with a connected series of rotational movements across multiple adjoining body segments and joints that combine into larger movement. Running is done mainly in the sagittal plane (see p.10). Rotations in this plane produce the forward-backward swinging of the arms and legs. In the transverse plane, the chest and pelvis segments move in alternating counter-rotation to each other.

WEATHER

There are many things you can control in your training and racing, but the weather is not one of them, and it can significantly impact your performance. Some climactic conditions can even lead to medical emergencies. However, with preparation and strategy adjustments, you can perform well in challenging weather conditions.

Heat

Exercising in the heat increases the perception of effort, meaning movement feels more challenging than in cooler conditions. This is possibly a biological safety mechanism that discourages us from pushing too hard in difficult conditions. To dissipate body heat in high temperatures, the body shunts blood away from the muscles and toward the skin (see pp.44–45). This decrease in oxygen supply to the muscles induces fatigue.

Using the heat

Training in the heat offers advantages. Heat is sometimes referred to as "the poor man's altitude" because training in hot conditions can have effects similar to those of altitude training (see opposite). The body adapts to the heat by increasing blood plasma volume, which allows greater capacity for carrying red blood cells to your working muscles. As little as 10 days of training in the heat has been shown to boost VO_2 max values by 5 percent.

Wind

The effect of overcoming wind resistance depends on the speed at which you are traveling. This is why wind speed is measured at sprint events and why cyclists race in packs, drafting off one another to save energy. The effect is less pronounced in endurance running, but research suggests that running economy improves while drafting behind someone, especially when running into a headwind.

DRAG

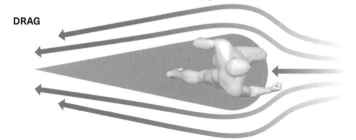

DRAFTING

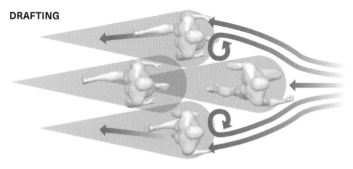

DRAG AND DRAFTING

The front-runners in this pack push through the air, diverting the air stream around them, creating turbulence and a pocket of negative air pressure behind them. Running within this pocket, the slipstream, reduces drag on the runner behind, who then requires less effort to run at the same pace as the others.

Humidity

Humidity impairs the body's ability to lose heat through sweating, which can significantly affect your heat tolerance. One useful tool is the wet-bulb globe temperature, a method for measuring temperature which factors in humidity, solar radiation, wind movement, and ambient temperature to estimate the sum effect of these climactic conditions on the human body. Many racing-event organizations now use this tool, along with the American College of Sports Medicine Heat and Humidity Guidelines for Races, to determine how safe it is to run on a given day. If you regularly train in hot and humid conditions, make use of WBGT readings to help you train safely.

Rain

While rain can make it difficult to get out the door at times, once you are outside, it is often quite refreshing and pleasant to be running in the rain. It can also help keep you cool and comfortable once you are warmed up. The danger comes when conditions are cold as well as wet, because once you are wet, your body finds it more difficult to retain heat, which can lead to hypothermia and other cold-related conditions. Investing in a good running jacket and wearing a hat and gloves can make a big difference to your safety in cold and wet conditions.

Cold

As you might expect, running in the cold produces the opposite physiological response to running in the heat. Blood is shunted away from the peripheries in order to retain heat. If training in cold conditions, dress appropriately. Select polyester clothing that wicks away sweat, and wear gloves and a warm hat to reduce heat loss from the extremities.

Air pollution

Air pollution is a concern for many runners living in large urban areas. There are several considerations when it comes to running in air-polluted zones. The amount of time you are exposed to pollution prerun matters. Driving for an hour through the city to go for a run indoors may not be worthwhile. Shorter, more intense workouts may be effective to minimize overall exposure. Running in the early morning or late evening, when pollution levels are generally lowest, is advisable. Give yourself some distance from active pollution—even small distances and barriers like trees can make a big difference. The decline in pollution levels as you move away from a road is exponential. Indoors is not always better—for instance, chemicals found in cleaning solutions and new carpets or furniture can compromise air quality. If you live in an area with high levels of air pollution, focus on the big picture as you weigh up your options: even exposure to high levels of traffic-related pollution does not outweigh the beneficial effects of physical activity.

TERRAIN

Different types of terrain present the runner's body with specific challenges. It takes practice to become proficient at running up and down hills. Likewise, running on uneven surfaces requires different types of muscle actions and carries specific injury risks. Running at altitude, of course, can make even an easy jog feel like a maximal effort.

Hills

Running uphill requires the body to overcome greater resistance than if running on the flat. You recruit more muscle fibers to power your center of mass off the ground and receive less contribution from the elastic recoil of tendons (see p.17), so more concentric muscle action (see p.19) is required. Gravity provides momentum when running downhill, but the impact forces experienced are greater, necessitating more eccentric muscle action (see p.18).

Variable surfaces

Running on a firm, even surface like a road or treadmill can produce fast, consistent results but may increase risk of overuse injury. Conversely, running on variable terrain such as trails will increase stride-to-stride variability (in cadence, footstrike, and so on), which can affect pace and running economy but can reduce the risk of overuse injury. Factors such as snow, ice, or loose gravel can also affect performance and change the muscle requirements.

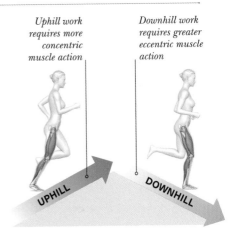

Uphill work requires more concentric muscle action

Downhill work requires greater eccentric muscle action

UPHILL

DOWNHILL

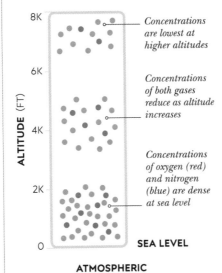

Concentrations are lowest at higher altitudes

Concentrations of both gases reduce as altitude increases

Concentrations of oxygen (red) and nitrogen (blue) are dense at sea level

ALTITUDE (FT)

8K

6K

4K

2K

0

SEA LEVEL

ATMOSPHERIC CONCENTRATION OF GASES

Altitude

Due to lower air pressure, being at altitude means there is less oxygen in the air available to be diffused into the blood. The lower blood oxygenation corresponds with a reduction in VO_2 max (see p.37). The effects of altitude can be felt as low as 1,900 ft (600 m) above sea level, although most runners are not affected until around 2,900 ft (900 m). Training at altitude produces a beneficial adaptation—it triggers an increase in the number of red blood cells that deliver oxygen to muscles. Consequently, many elite athletes travel to high altitudes to train before racing at sea level.

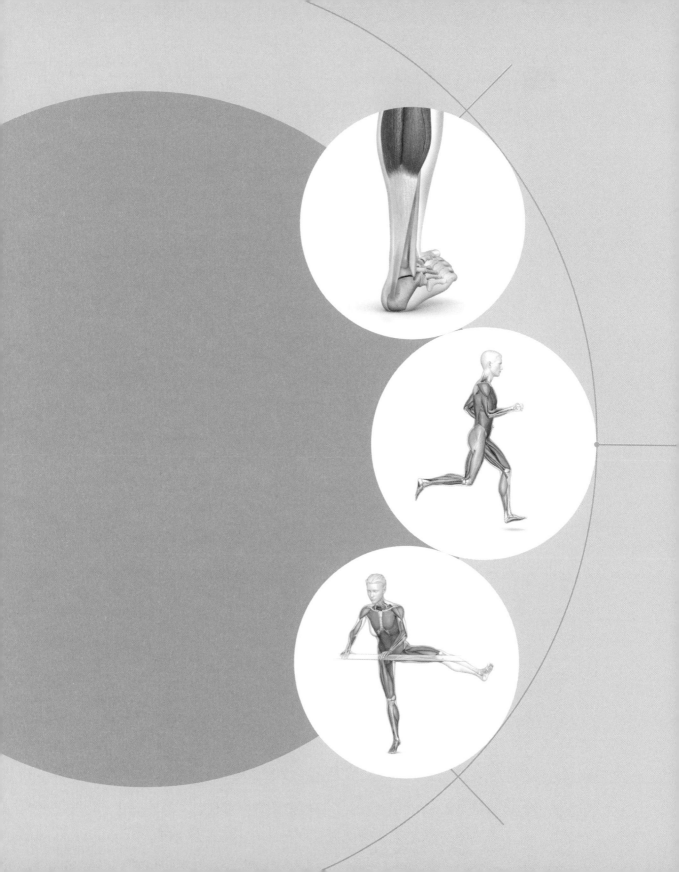

PREVENTING INJURY

Every runner knows that injuries are part of the sport, but also knows too well how frustrating it feels to be unable to run. A little education can go a long way toward preventing injuries in the first place and speeding recovery from injuries when they do happen. This chapter explains how injuries occur and outlines ways in which you can minimize your own specific risk.

INJURY **RISKS**

There are numerous health benefits to running, but it also carries an inherent risk of injury. Most injuries result from overuse rather than trauma. Broadly speaking, there are three main categories of risk considered to cause running injuries: biomechanical factors, anatomical factors, and training error.

UP TO
50%
OF RUNNERS
EXPERIENCE A
RUNNING INJURY
EACH YEAR

BIOMECHANICAL
FACTORS

A runner's biomechanics—how they move and position different parts of their body as they run—is known as "running form," and your individual form can have an effect on your risk of injury. Several common injuries, such as patellofemoral pain, iliotibial band pain, and stress fractures of the tibia, have been linked to specific running biomechanics.

Recent research suggests that improving your running form may help protect against injury. Learn all about running biomechanics and how to assess and make changes to your running form on pp.66–75.

ANATOMICAL
FACTORS

Some anatomical "abnormalities," such as flat feet or knock knees, are considered risk factors for running injuries, but this belief has not been backed up by research. Your body becomes accustomed to its own anatomy and will adapt to your training as long as you build up your training load gradually.

TRAINING
ERROR

Fluctuations in your training load are a common mistake. Running repeatedly subjects the body to impact forces (see pp.46–47), causing tissue breakdown that requires time to heal. When you overtrain, the repair process cannot keep pace with the rate at which those stresses are being applied, leading to injury.

INJURY **SITES**

Most running-related injuries affect the lower body. The most common site of injury is the knee, followed by the ankle and foot. However, depending on your running biomechanics, you may be prone to some injuries more than others (see opposite). Injury sites also depend on sex, with females tending to suffer a greater proportion of knee injuries than males.

LOCATING INJURY RISK
Almost one-third of all running injuries occur at the knee, followed closely by the ankle, foot, and shinbone. Female runners are at greater risk of knee and hip injury, while male runners are more prone to issues involving the shinbone and ankle or foot.

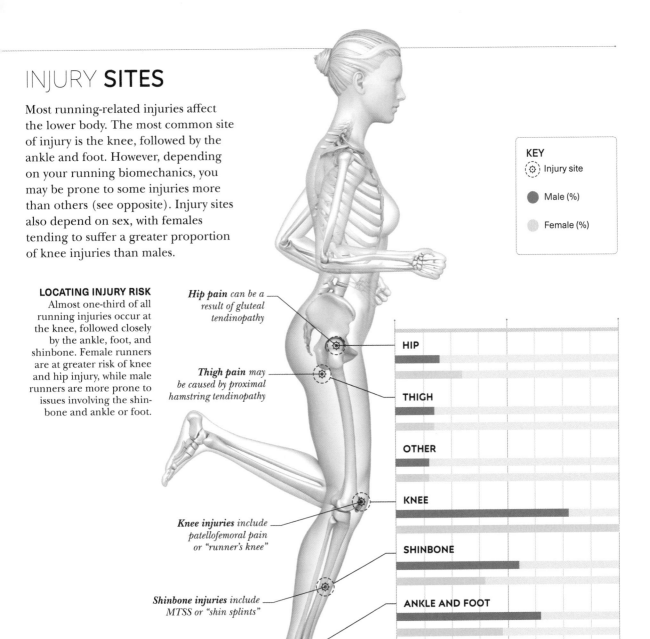

KEY
⊙ Injury site
● Male (%)
● Female (%)

Hip pain can be a result of gluteal tendinopathy

Thigh pain may be caused by proximal hamstring tendinopathy

Knee injuries include patellofemoral pain or "runner's knee"

Shinbone injuries include MTSS or "shin splints"

Ankle and foot injuries include plantar heel pain and Achilles tendinopathy

HIP

THIGH

OTHER

KNEE

SHINBONE

ANKLE AND FOOT

0   20   40

RUNNING-RELATED INJURIES BY SITE:
COMPARING MEN AND WOMEN (%)

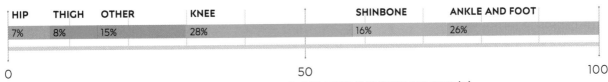

HIP	THIGH	OTHER	KNEE	SHINBONE	ANKLE AND FOOT
7%	8%	15%	28%	16%	26%

0   50   100

PERCENTAGE OF RUNNING-RELATED INJURIES BY SITE (%)

COMMON INJURIES

The risk of injury is part of the sport of running, and unfortunately many runners experience the injuries described on the following pages. However, armed with a little knowledge, there are things you can do to maximize your chances of complete recovery should you get injured.

WHEN TO STOP TRAINING

Runners are known for running through pain, but it is crucial to recognize the difference between the pain of exertion and the pain of injury. If you feel pain that you would rate greater than 3/10 (see right) during or after a run, stop training and seek advice from a physical therapist. Another signal to stop is if your running gait changes due to pain. Some wearable sensors can detect asymmetries early on to warn of potential changes in gait.

Rating your pain

Nonlocalized stiffness and mild pain are to be expected after a workout, but pain registering as moderate or above could indicate injury.

Assess any pain you feel on a scale of 1 to 10

MILD MODERATE SEVERE VERY SEVERE

NONE ────────────── WORST

0 1 2 3 4 5 6 7 8 9 10

PAIN SCALE

LIGAMENT GRAFT — 2 MONTHS–1 YEAR
ARTICULAR CARTILAGE REPAIR — 2 MONTHS–1 YEAR
LIGAMENT SPRAIN: GRADE 3 — 5 WEEKS–1 YEAR
GRADE 2 — 3 WEEKS–6 MONTHS
GRADE 1 — 0–3 DAYS
TENDON: TENDINITIS — 3 WEEKS–7 WEEKS
TENDINOSIS — 3 MONTHS–6 MONTHS
LACERATION — 5 WEEKS–6 MONTHS
MUSCLE STRAIN: GRADE 3 — 3 WEEKS–6 MONTHS
GRADE 2 — 4 DAYS–3 MONTHS
GRADE 1 — 0–2 WEEKS
BONE — 5 WEEKS–3 MONTHS
MUSCLE SORENESS POSTEXERCISE — 0–3 DAYS

SELF-HELP

Think POLICE to remember the self-help measures you can take if you suffer injury:

- **Protection:** Protect the injured area by taping or wearing a brace or by using off-the-shelf orthotics to redistribute pressure from the site.
- **Optimal (and early) Loading:** Do not overwork injured tissue, but don't avoid using it either. Keep moving to maintain strength and range of movement. Pain-avoidance movement patterns can become habitual, which may affect your running gait and lead to further injury.
- **Ice:** Apply ice to the injured site for pain relief.
- **Compression and Elevation:** Elevate the injured site and use compression bandages or socks to reduce swelling and limit tissue damage.

INJURY HEALING TIMES
Differences in blood supply and cellular turnover mean some tissues take longer than others to heal. Bear this in mind when returning to training. While you may feel healed, some tissues may not yet be ready for a more challenging training load.

PATELLOFEMORAL PAIN

Also known as "runner's knee," this condition is experienced as pain around, behind, or under the patella (kneecap). Pain can range from mild to severe and may be felt during a run or while performing day-to-day activities such as walking, sitting, squatting, or climbing stairs.

COMMON CAUSES

Patellofemoral pain has many causes. Not all of them are running-related, but excessive or rapid increases in training often contribute. Individual biomechanics, such as increased hip adduction (see p.10), may also be a risk factor, as can running on harder surfaces and downhill running.

TREATMENT

Seek help early for the best chance of recovery. Treatment can include:
- Short-term pain reduction through taping, bracing, and the use of off-the-shelf orthotics.
- A temporary reduction in your training load.
- Professional gait retraining may help if you have a biomechanical risk factor.
- Following a program of static stretches and strength exercises that target the hip and thigh muscles: see pp.92–93, 118–129, and 136–139.

RETURNING TO TRAINING

Recovery time will vary; use pain as a guide for when to return to training. Low-impact cross-training on a stationary bike or in the pool will help maintain fitness while building up strength. Increase your training load gradually and stick to running on softer surfaces and avoiding hills to reaccustom the knee to impact. If you usually run on roads or a treadmill, try trails, which have more variable terrain.

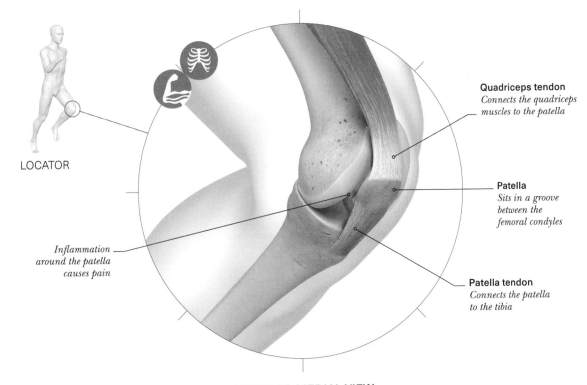

LOCATOR

Quadriceps tendon
Connects the quadriceps muscles to the patella

Patella
Sits in a groove between the femoral condyles

Patella tendon
Connects the patella to the tibia

Inflammation around the patella causes pain

ANTERIOR-MEDIAL VIEW

ACHILLES TENDINOPATHY

This is a degenerative condition caused by structural changes to the tendon itself, which result in pain along the tendon or at its insertion onto the heel bone. The heel may feel painful in the morning or at the start of a run, but symptoms may subside once warmed up. The condition can become a chronic and disabling injury if it isn't dealt with quickly and appropriately.

COMMON CAUSES

Achilles tendinopathy usually develops because of a rapid increase in your training load (whether distance, frequency, or intensity) or due to individual biomechanics, changes in footwear, or running on harder terrain.

TREATMENT

Early treatment offers the best chance of full recovery and can include the following:

- Anti-inflammatory medication for pain relief, if needed.
- A temporary reduction in your training load.
- Wearing shoes with higher heels or wedges to unload the tendon.
- A program of dynamic calf stretches and strength training for the Achilles tendon: see pp. 82–83, 108–111, and 154–155.

RETURNING TO TRAINING

If the condition is recognized early, reducing your training load could settle the Achilles tendon in 5–10 days. Once the tendon has settled, gradually bring your training load back up to previous levels. Bear in mind that pain is not always a good indicator in tendon injuries, as it may take up to 24 hours to feel symptoms if you've overloaded the tendon. Low-impact cross-training in the pool or on the bike will help maintain fitness while building up strength. Speed work and running uphill can place stress on the tendon and are best avoided until the condition has healed.

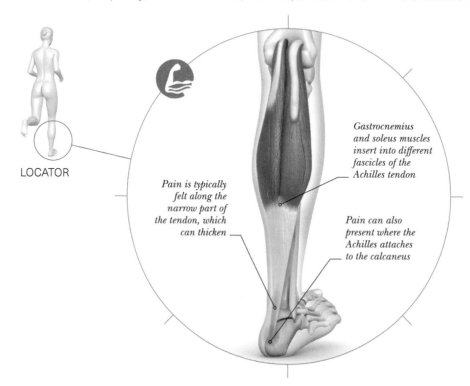

LOCATOR

Pain is typically felt along the narrow part of the tendon, which can thicken

Gastrocnemius and soleus muscles insert into different fascicles of the Achilles tendon

Pain can also present where the Achilles attaches to the calcaneus

POSTERIOR-LATERAL VIEW

MEDIAL TIBIAL STRESS SYNDROME (MTSS)

Often called "shin splints," MTSS causes mild to severe pain along the inside of the tibia (shinbone) during weight-bearing exercise. The affected area is usually tender when touched and spans at least 2 in (5 cm). MTSS is common in new runners but can also occur after running on a different surface, using new shoes, or increasing your training intensity.

COMMON CAUSES

Increased impact forces on the body often bring on MTSS, caused by running on harder or cambered surfaces, or the cumulative impact from a sudden increase in your training load. Some biomechanical risk factors, such as increased pronation (see p.73) or abduction, narrow step width (see p.71), or lower cadence (<170 steps/min; see p.70), may also cause MTSS.

TREATMENT

No single treatment is effective, but the following should help:
- A temporary reduction in your training load.
- A program of graded loading exposure (incremental increases to your training load) can help manage the toll of impact forces, taking into account your training history, surface, and footwear.
- Gait retraining may help if you have a biomechanical risk factor.
- Strength training for the soleus and tibialis posterior: see pp.108–111 and 112–117.

RETURNING TO TRAINING

If treated early, recovery can be quick; use pain as a guide for when to increase your training. Low-impact cross-training in the pool or on the bike will help maintain fitness. Rebuild impact tolerance by increasing your training load gradually, ideally running on softer terrain (such as trails) and avoiding cambered surfaces or running down hills.

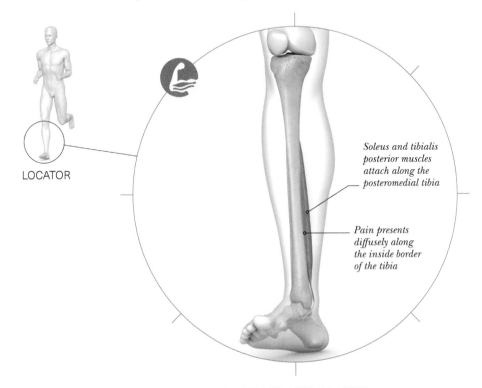

LOCATOR

Soleus and tibialis posterior muscles attach along the posteromedial tibia

Pain presents diffusely along the inside border of the tibia

ANTERIOR–MEDIAL VIEW

PLANTAR HEEL PAIN

This covers several conditions affecting the underside of the heel, the most common being plantar fasciitis. Typically, pain is felt when bearing weight on the heel, especially in the morning and after periods of inactivity, but may subside while running. The area can be extremely tender to the touch.

COMMON CAUSES

Plantar heel pain usually develops because of a rapid increase in your training load (distance, frequency, or intensity), from running on hard terrain, wearing new or unsuitable footwear (both running and casual), or as a result of individual biomechanical risk factors.

TREATMENT

Seek help early to improve your chances of recovery with the following treatments:

- Wearing supportive shoes or off-the-shelf orthotics to distribute pressure away from the heel in order to settle the pain initially. Introduce new shoes gradually by rotating them with old ones.
- A temporary reduction in your training load.
- A program of calf stretches and strength exercises targeting the plantar fascia and intrinsic foot muscles: see pp.82–83, 100–107, and 110–111.

RETURNING TO TRAINING

Severity and duration of pain influences recovery time. If the plantar fascia is overloaded, it may take up to 24 hours to feel symptoms, meaning pain is not always a good indicator for judging training load. Low-impact cross-training in the pool or on the bike helps maintain fitness while building up strength. Avoid speed work until fully healed.

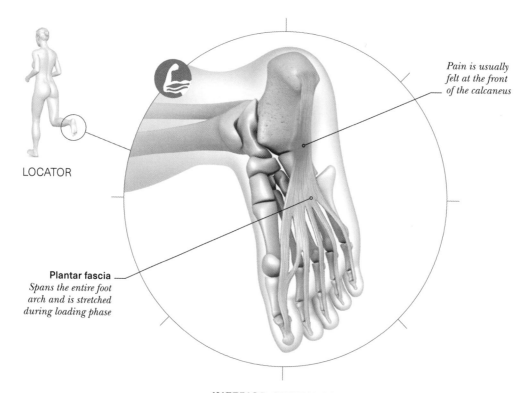

LOCATOR

Pain is usually felt at the front of the calcaneus

Plantar fascia
Spans the entire foot arch and is stretched during loading phase

INFERIOR-MEDIAL VIEW

ILIOTIBIAL BAND PAIN

The iliotibial (IT) band is a tendonlike structure that extends along the outside of the leg from the hip to the knee. The condition is felt as pain over the outside of the knee as it bends in midstance (see p.67). The pain can be sharp and debilitating and is often made worse with prolonged downhill running.

COMMON CAUSES

IT band pain often develops from a rapid increase in training, especially if it features downhill running. Some biomechanical risk factors can also put strain on the IT band.

These include contralateral pelvic drop (see p.73), increased hip adduction (see p.10), and narrow step width (see p.71). The pain is thought to be due to compression of structures deep to the IT band and not from the band itself.

TREATMENT

The following treatments may be recommended:
- Strength training for the hip abductors: see pp.118–131 and 136–139.
- Dynamic and recovery stretches, including a stretch to release the tensor fasciae latae (TFL)

muscles (the IT band itself cannot be stretched or released): see pp.78–79 and 90–95.
- Reduction in your training load by decreasing volume and avoiding downhill runs.
- Gait retraining may help those with a biomechanical risk factor.

RETURNING TO TRAINING

Recovery time depends on the duration of the IT band pain. Do not run through the pain; limit your runs to distances that are pain-free. Runners who return to high-volume training too soon often reaggravate the injury.

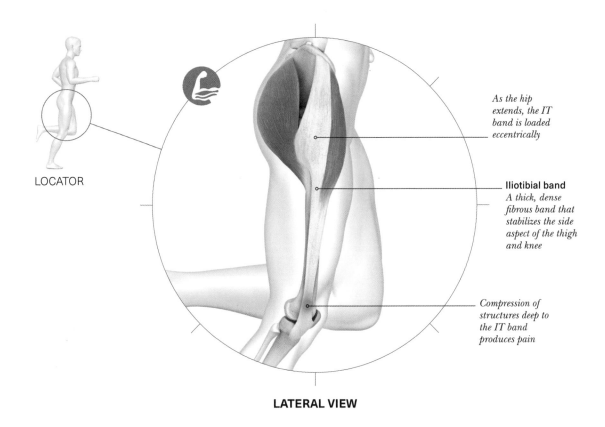

LOCATOR

As the hip extends, the IT band is loaded eccentrically

Iliotibial band
A thick, dense fibrous band that stabilizes the side aspect of the thigh and knee

Compression of structures deep to the IT band produces pain

LATERAL VIEW

DEEP GLUTEAL SYNDROME

Previously known as piriformis syndrome, this condition describes buttock pain caused by trapping or compression of the sciatic nerve within the hip. Pain is felt deep in the buttock and may be accompanied by sciatic pain or cramping along the back of the thigh. Long periods of running and sitting can aggravate it.

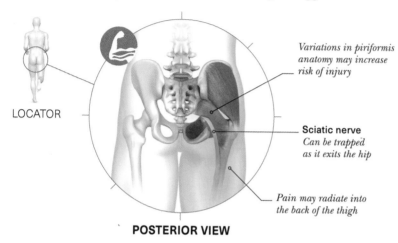

LOCATOR

Variations in piriformis anatomy may increase risk of injury

Sciatic nerve
Can be trapped as it exits the hip

Pain may radiate into the back of the thigh

POSTERIOR VIEW

COMMON CAUSES
Deep gluteal syndrome usually develops after significant increases in running duration or intensity. In many cases, it is preceded by some sort of lower back pain or trauma, such as from a fall or childbirth.

TREATMENT
The following actions may be recommended to aid recovery:
- Reducing your time spent sitting.
- Sciatic "flossing" (nerve stretching) exercises combined with the manipulation and kneading of the muscles by a physical therapist.
- A graded program of strength-training exercises targeting muscles of the hip abductors,

GLUTEAL TENDINOPATHY

Often referred to as greater trochanteric bursitis, gluteal tendinopathy is pain and tenderness felt in the side of the hip where the gluteal tendon attaches to the top of the femur. Symptoms are often disabling since it can be uncomfortable to run, walk, or even lie on the affected side.

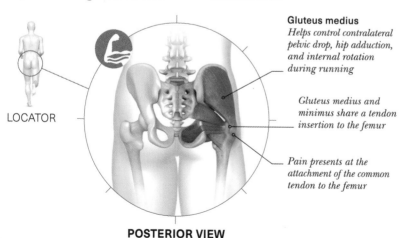

LOCATOR

Gluteus medius
Helps control contralateral pelvic drop, hip adduction, and internal rotation during running

Gluteus medius and minimus share a tendon insertion to the femur

Pain presents at the attachment of the common tendon to the femur

POSTERIOR VIEW

COMMON CAUSES
Gluteal tendinopathy is caused by repetitive stress on the gluteal tendon. Impact forces absorbed by the leg as the foot strikes the ground (see pp.66–67) can damage the tendon if it cannot cope with the rate of the load applied. Downhill running and biomechanical factors, such as increased hip adduction (see p.10) and knee valgus (see p.73), can also lead to this injury.

TREATMENT
The following actions may be recommended to aid recovery:
- For those with a biomechanical risk factor, professional gait retraining may be useful.

extensors, and external rotators to increase their ability to support the loads related to running: see pp.118–119, 122–131, and 136–139.

- Dynamic and static stretching, particularly of the back of the hip to relieve tension on the nerve: see pp.78–83 and 90–95.

RETURNING TO TRAINING

Reduce your training load, but do not stop running altogether. Avoid longer runs, speed work, and running uphill initially. Spend more time on your dynamic warm-up—especially forward leg swing (see pp.78–79) and side leg swing (see pp.80–81)—to increase the range of motion at the hip.

- Recovery stretches for the back of the hip: see pp.90–95.
- Strength exercises for the hip abductor muscles: see pp.118–131, 136–139, and 142–143.

RETURNING TO TRAINING

Reduce your training load, but don't stop running altogether. Increase load gradually as symptoms allow. Bear in mind, pain is not always a good indicator in tendon injuries, as it may take up to 24 hours to feel symptoms if the tendon has been overloaded. Low-impact cross-training in the pool or on the bike will help maintain fitness while building up strength. Try running on softer ground and avoid speed work and downhill running.

STRESS FRACTURE

Stress fractures are fatigue-induced cracks in the bone that develop due to overtraining and inadequate rest. Runners most commonly suffer stress fractures in the shinbone, foot, hip, and sacrum (lower back bone).

COMMON CAUSES

Cumulative overload is the main cause, often when the volume or intensity of your training suddenly increases. Running with a forefoot strike pattern (see p.72) has also been linked to fractures in the metatarsals due to the higher loads in this area. Poor nutrition and hormonal status can lead to an elevated risk of stress fracture and overall reduced bone health. Long-term energy deficits may lead to a condition known as Relative Energy Deficiency in Sport (RED-S).

TREATMENT

Stop running, reduce weight bearing, and seek help early:

- Rest is the main treatment for a stress fracture.
- Depending on the stage and severity of the fracture, it can be beneficial to resume weight bearing early, sometimes in an orthotic boot, to maintain bone mass and strength.

RETURNING TO TRAINING

Following a stress fracture, it is vital to build up your training load gradually and progressively. A walk-run program is usually recommended to reintroduce the impact to your body. You should be able to hop for 30 seconds pain-free each day for a week before resuming any running training.

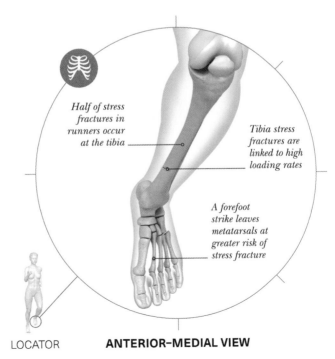

Half of stress fractures in runners occur at the tibia

Tibia stress fractures are linked to high loading rates

A forefoot strike leaves metatarsals at greater risk of stress fracture

LOCATOR **ANTERIOR-MEDIAL VIEW**

AVOIDING INJURY

Most runners get injured from time to time, but there are things you can do to lower your injury risk. Be aware of your running biomechanics, keep an eye on your body's response to training, incorporate strength exercises into your training regime, and know when to seek help.

PRINCIPLES OF INJURY PREVENTION

Following some basic principles can help you run pain-free and may improve performance.

CONSIDER BIOMECHANICS

Our individual running form makes each of us more prone to certain injuries. For example, if you strike the ground with the forefoot rather than the heel, impact force increases at the calf. Assess your form for injury risk and make any necessary improvements (see pp.66–75).

MONITOR TRAINING LOAD

Spikes in your training load are the main cause of injury, so it's vital to increase your training gradually. Both the volume and intensity of training affect the toll on your body; digital tracking tools can be used to monitor load (see pp.168–169).

DO STRENGTH EXERCISES

Strengthening muscles and joints through resistance training (see pp.97–155) improves your body's

ability to handle your training load and has been shown to improve performance. A runner should opt for higher resistance and lower reps in a strength-training session.

SEEK PROFESSIONAL HELP

If you experience pain rated as greater than 3 out of 10 (see p.56), if your gait changes as a result of pain, or if your pain is worsening, seek advice from a clinician who is familiar with running.

Footwear and injury prevention

Despite the huge sums of money spent by footwear companies on research and development, neither traditional running shoes nor recent minimalist and maximalist designs have been proven to prevent injury.

Minimalist shoes, for instance, are claimed to help increase running cadence, alter footstrike patterns, and reduce vertical loading rates. However, in the most comprehensive study conducted to date, stride parameters and footstrike patterns remained unchanged after a 6-month transition to minimalist footwear, and there are also conflicting findings on the effect of minimalist shoes on loading rates.

As far as performance is concerned, it is accepted that lighter is better. For every 3½ oz (100 g) of weight added, your running economy worsens by around 1 percent. Carbon fiber plates and hyper-resilient foam have also been shown to improve running economy but at significant financial cost.

CHANGING SHOES
An abrupt change in cushioning or heel offset can result in injury. If moving to minimalist shoes, strengthen foot and calf muscles (see pp.100–111).

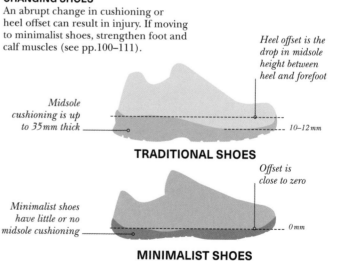

Heel offset is the drop in midsole height between heel and forefoot

Midsole cushioning is up to 35 mm thick

10–12 mm

TRADITIONAL SHOES

Offset is close to zero

Minimalist shoes have little or no midsole cushioning

0 mm

MINIMALIST SHOES

Special considerations

One of the greatest things about running as a sport is that almost anyone can take it up. Nonetheless, some runners should take special considerations into account in order to reduce their risk of injury.

FACTORS	RISKS	PREVENTION
AGE	Younger runners whose bodies are still maturing may be at greater risk of injury, especially bone and tendon injuries. Older runners are at increased risk of Achilles and calf injuries due to decreased strength and changes in biomechanics.	Younger runners should be careful with their training load, erring on the low side. Older runners should include strength-based exercises (see pp.96–155) and pay attention to running form (see pp.66–75).
SEX	Masculine and feminine body types have different injury risk profiles. Studies show that feminine physiques are more prone to knee injuries and a masculine physique can suffer more ankle, foot, and shinbone injuries. It is not clear which physical type is injured more frequently.	Targeted strength training (see pp.96–155) and also improvements in running form (see pp.66–75) can help reduce injury risk for all runners, regardless of sex-based physique.
EXCESS WEIGHT	Overweight runners are subjected to greater impact forces per step. Cumulatively, these impacts may increase risk of injury.	Be careful not to increase your training load too quickly, and allow time for your musculoskeletal system to adapt to the loads applied.
PREGNANCY	Physical exercise during pregnancy is beneficial for most women, but there are some increased risk factors for pregnant runners due to hormonal changes, stress on the pelvic floor, and fatigue.	Follow the latest antenatal exercise guidelines and consult your physician or midwife before commencing or continuing any exercise program.
POSTPARTUM	After giving birth, women may be at greater risk of pelvic floor dysfunction, musculo-skeletal injuries, and Relative Energy Deficiency in Sport (RED-S; see p.63).	New mothers should wait 3 months and should be assessed by a pelvic health therapist before returning to running. Follow a graded return to running, such as a walk-run program (see pp.190–191).

*Adding **strength exercises** to your training regime improves the capacity of your **musculoskeletal system** to handle running loads*

RUNNING **CYCLE**

Running can be understood as a cycle of two main phases of movement—stance and swing—punctuated by certain key events (see pp.14–15). Most injury occurs during stance phase, and it is worth examining its subphases in detail to better appreciate the loads to which a runner is subjected.

EARLY LOADING PHASE

As the leading foot makes initial contact with the ground, the body decelerates in the vertical direction and significant muscle contributions are needed to control and attenuate the ground reaction force (GRF). As the foot flattens, tendons and connective tissues within muscles store elastic energy to be used later for propulsion.

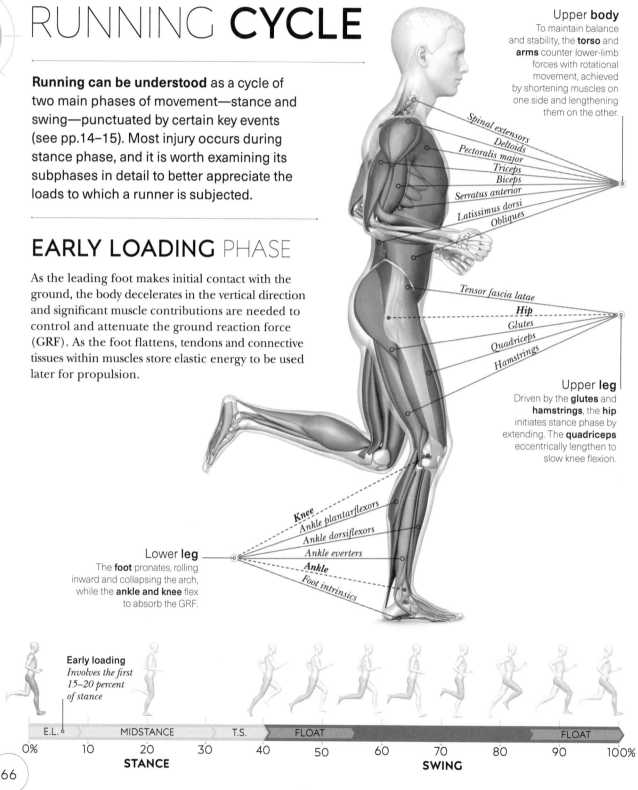

Upper **body**
To maintain balance and stability, the **torso** and **arms** counter lower-limb forces with rotational movement, achieved by shortening muscles on one side and lengthening them on the other.

Spinal extensors
Deltoids
Pectoralis major
Triceps
Biceps
Serratus anterior
Latissimus dorsi
Obliques

Tensor fascia latae
Hip
Glutes
Quadriceps
Hamstrings

Upper **leg**
Driven by the **glutes** and **hamstrings**, the **hip** initiates stance phase by extending. The **quadriceps** eccentrically lengthen to slow knee flexion.

Knee
Ankle plantarflexors
Ankle dorsiflexors
Ankle everters
Ankle
Foot intrinsics

Lower **leg**
The **foot** pronates, rolling inward and collapsing the arch, while the **ankle and knee** flex to absorb the GRF.

Early loading
Involves the first 15–20 percent of stance

E.L.	MIDSTANCE	T.S.	FLOAT	FLOAT

0%   10   20   30   40   50   60   70   80   90   100%

STANCE　　　　　　**SWING**

MIDSTANCE PHASE

In midstance, the body transitions from absorbing GRF to releasing recycled GRF energy. As the body passes over the top of the supporting leg, it must be dynamically stabilized to cope with maximal loading through the limb.

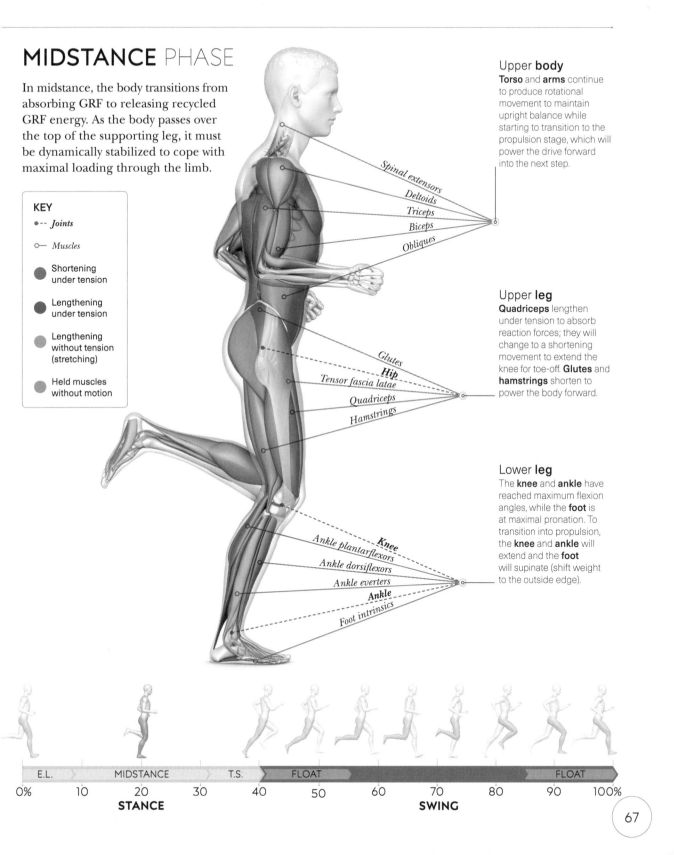

KEY

•--- *Joints*

○— *Muscles*

● Shortening under tension

● Lengthening under tension

● Lengthening without tension (stretching)

● Held muscles without motion

Spinal extensors
Deltoids
Triceps
Biceps
Obliques

Glutes
Hip
Tensor fascia latae
Quadriceps
Hamstrings

Knee
Ankle plantarflexors
Ankle dorsiflexors
Ankle everters
Ankle
Foot intrinsics

Upper **body**

Torso and **arms** continue to produce rotational movement to maintain upright balance while starting to transition to the propulsion stage, which will power the drive forward into the next step.

Upper **leg**

Quadriceps lengthen under tension to absorb reaction forces; they will change to a shortening movement to extend the knee for toe-off. **Glutes** and **hamstrings** shorten to power the body forward.

Lower **leg**

The **knee** and **ankle** have reached maximum flexion angles, while the **foot** is at maximal pronation. To transition into propulsion, the **knee** and **ankle** will extend and the **foot** will supinate (shift weight to the outside edge).

| E.L. | MIDSTANCE | T.S. | FLOAT | | FLOAT |

0% — 10 — 20 — 30 — 40 — 50 — 60 — 70 — 80 — 90 — 100%

STANCE   **SWING**

TERMINAL STANCE PHASE

This final subphase culminates in toe-off, when the hip, knee, and ankle are in maximal extension to propel the body forward. Immediately after toe-off, the hip and knee begin to move into flexion and the ankle starts to dorsiflex, preparing for the swing phase.

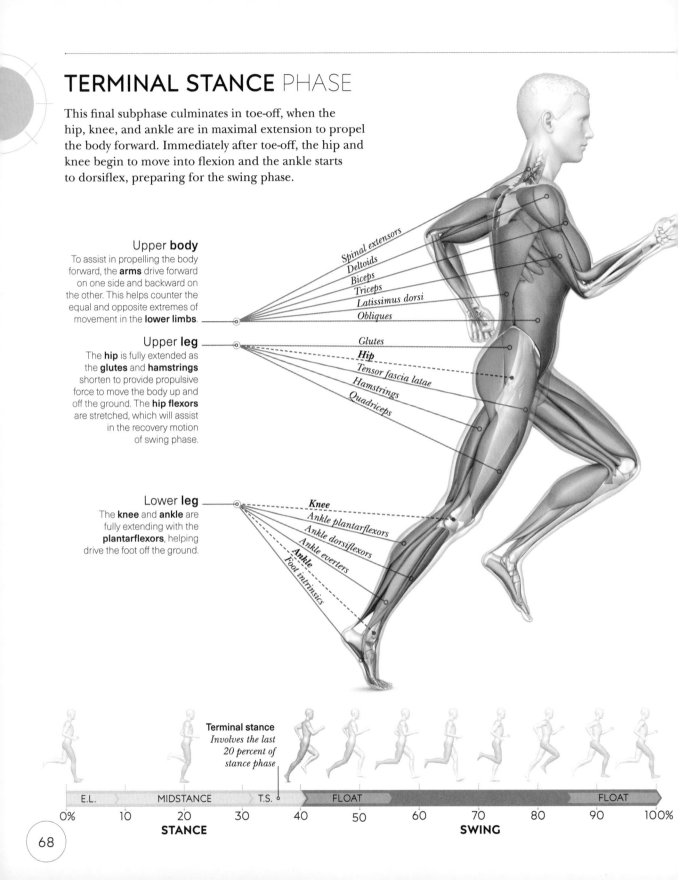

Upper **body**
To assist in propelling the body forward, the **arms** drive forward on one side and backward on the other. This helps counter the equal and opposite extremes of movement in the **lower limbs**.

Spinal extensors
Deltoids
Biceps
Triceps
Latissimus dorsi
Obliques

Upper **leg**
The **hip** is fully extended as the **glutes** and **hamstrings** shorten to provide propulsive force to move the body up and off the ground. The **hip flexors** are stretched, which will assist in the recovery motion of swing phase.

Glutes
Hip
Tensor fascia latae
Hamstrings
Quadriceps

Lower **leg**
The **knee** and **ankle** are fully extending with the **plantarflexors**, helping drive the foot off the ground.

Knee
Ankle plantarflexors
Ankle dorsiflexors
Ankle everters
Ankle
Foot intrinsics

Terminal stance
Involves the last 20 percent of stance phase

| E.L. | MIDSTANCE | T.S. | FLOAT | | FLOAT |

0%   10   20   30   40   50   60   70   80   90   100%

STANCE | **SWING**

SWING PHASE

Comprising approximately 60 percent of the running cycle, swing phase is when the hip flexes rapidly to swing the leg through until it recovers its starting position, ready to power another step. During late swing, the knee begins to extend and prepare again for stance.

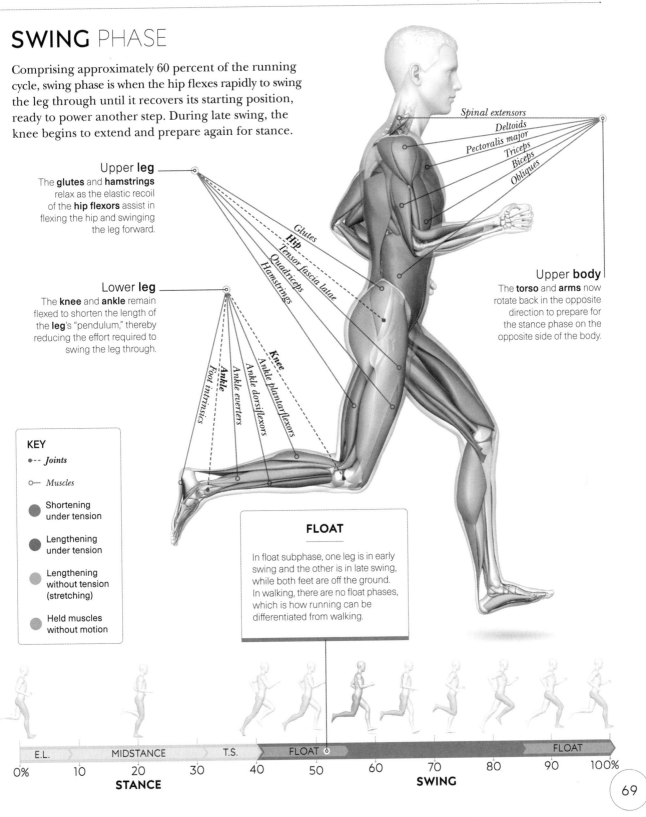

Spinal extensors
Deltoids
Pectoralis major
Triceps
Biceps
Obliques

Upper **leg**
The **glutes** and **hamstrings** relax as the elastic recoil of the **hip flexors** assist in flexing the hip and swinging the leg forward.

Lower **leg**
The **knee** and **ankle** remain flexed to shorten the length of the **leg**'s "pendulum," thereby reducing the effort required to swing the leg through.

Glutes
Hip
Tensor fascia latae
Quadriceps
Hamstrings

Knee
Ankle plantarflexors
Ankle dorsiflexors
Ankle everters
Ankle
Foot intrinsics

Upper **body**
The **torso** and **arms** now rotate back in the opposite direction to prepare for the stance phase on the opposite side of the body.

KEY

●--- *Joints*

○— *Muscles*

● Shortening under tension

● Lengthening under tension

● Lengthening without tension (stretching)

● Held muscles without motion

FLOAT

In float subphase, one leg is in early swing and the other is in late swing, while both feet are off the ground. In walking, there are no float phases, which is how running can be differentiated from walking.

E.L.	MIDSTANCE		T.S.	FLOAT ○			FLOAT
0%	10	20	30	40	50	60	70	80	90	100%
	STANCE						**SWING**			

INDIVIDUAL GAIT

No running gait is perfect, but it may be worth adjusting your gait to increase efficiency or help avoid injury, especially one that is recurring. If you identify an issue, consult a health professional or coach who can offer safe ways to help change your gait.

STRIDE PATTERN

If you have been told you land heavily or look inefficient when you run, you may need to adjust your stride. An ideal stride is one that allows you to move forward with as little braking or bouncing as possible.

Overstriding

If your feet each tend to land too far in front of you when making initial contact (see pp.14 and 66), this is known as overstriding and causes increased braking forces. These forces reduce running efficiency and increase stress to the shinbone, knee, hip, and lower back.

Increasing cadence

A safe and effective way to eliminate overstriding is to increase your step rate, or "cadence." This reduces your step length and causes your foot to land closer to your center of mass. Increased cadence also reduces vertical and braking forces, gluteal demand, knee-joint loads, forces acting on the Achilles tendon, and vertical oscillation (see right). An increase in cadence of 5–10 percent is generally sufficient. A way to achieve this is to run with a metronome set to your goal cadence. These can be downloaded onto your phone or set to beep on your running watch.

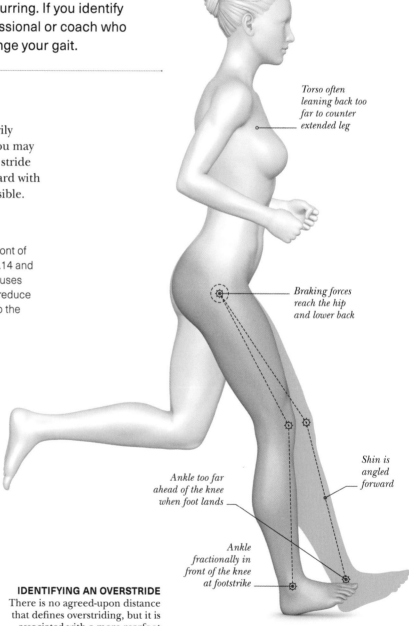

Torso often leaning back too far to counter extended leg

Braking forces reach the hip and lower back

Shin is angled forward

Ankle too far ahead of the knee when foot lands

Ankle fractionally in front of the knee at footstrike

IDENTIFYING AN OVERSTRIDE
There is no agreed-upon distance that defines overstriding, but it is associated with a more rearfoot strike and overextended knee.

LATERAL VIEW

Vertical oscillation

Some vertical oscillation is needed in running, but too much is a bad thing. Increased oscillation is linked to greater vertical loading and decreased running efficiency. There is no agreed ideal level of oscillation, but you can get a sense of how much you bounce by watching yourself run in a mirror or having someone film you. Ways to reduce vertical oscillation include trying to "land softly" or imagining you are running under a low ceiling. Increasing cadence also reduces vertical oscillation (see left).

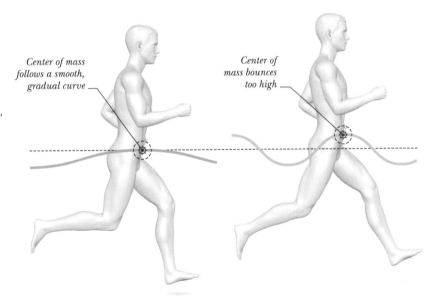

Center of mass follows a smooth, gradual curve

Center of mass bounces too high

EFFICIENT OSCILLATION
The center of mass does not bounce up and down to a significant degree from one step to the next. This is usually associated with a shorter stride and higher cadence.

EXCESSIVE OSCILLATION
The center of mass bounces up and down inefficiently from one step to the next. Energy is wasted propelling the center of mass upward against gravity instead of forward in the direction of travel.

Step width

The lateral alignment of the feet as they strike the ground is called step width. We step with a narrower gait when running than walking since it is more energy efficient. Taking narrow steps requires greater dynamic stability and strength in the hip abductors, which can pose an injury risk.

Running with knees apart

Increasing your step width may help if you suffer from conditions such as IT band pain, patellofemoral pain, or tibialis posterior tendon dysfunction. While it is difficult to identify where your feet line up as you run, one way that seems to work is to run with your knees apart. If you have a mirror in front of you or can be filmed from behind, you should be able to see a clear space between your knees throughout the running cycle.

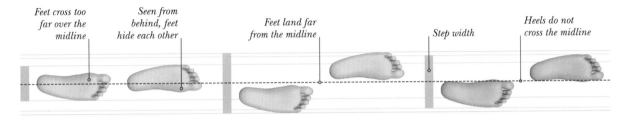

Feet cross too far over the midline

Seen from behind, feet hide each other

Feet land far from the midline

Step width

Heels do not cross the midline

NARROW STEP WIDTH
A narrow width increases the amount and velocity of pronation (see p.73) and increases strain on the lateral hip, associated with various injury risks (see box, left).

WIDE STEP WIDTH
A wider step increases the amount of energy expended in the running cycle, so there is a balance to be struck between injury reduction and an efficient gait.

EFFICIENT STEP WIDTH
You should be able to see daylight between your knees throughout the cycle. Seen from behind, the feet should not hide each other as one steps in front of the other.

FOOTSTRIKE PATTERNS

Footstrike refers to the point on your foot that first hits the ground
at initial contact (see pp.14 and 66). The notions that a rearfoot strike
increases injury risk and that a forefoot strike is more economical have both
been refuted by recent research. In reality, where you land simply shifts
the location of forces on your body during the loading phase. Depending
on your injury history, this may be an important consideration.

Rearfoot strike

Between 80 and 95 percent
of all distance runners are
rearfoot strikers who land on
the rear third of their foot at
initial contact. This is linked
to a more dorsiflexed ankle,
where the toes turn upward
toward the shin. A rearfoot
strike is associated with greater
vertical loading rates.

Knee subjected
to greater force

GRF passes
behind the
ankle joint

Reduced stress on
foot, ankle, and
calf muscles

Forefoot strike

Forefoot striking is defined
as landing on the front third
of your foot at initial contact.
This is associated with a
plantarflexed ankle, where the
toes point away from the shin.
A forefoot strike pattern is
believed to produce greater
braking forces.

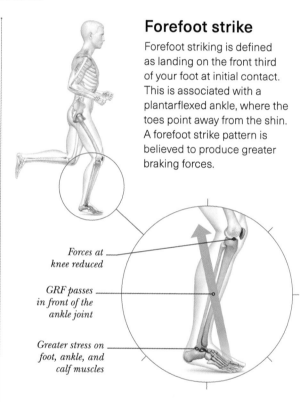

Forces at
knee reduced

GRF passes
in front of the
ankle joint

Greater stress on
foot, ankle, and
calf muscles

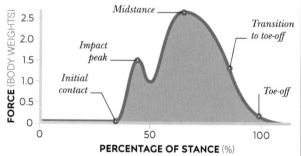

VERTICAL GRF WITH REARFOOT STRIKE
The rearfoot GRF (see pp.46–47) profile shows an
impact peak from the force of the foot hitting the
ground. The force direction reduces load on Achilles
tendon but increases it on tibialis anterior muscle.

VERTICAL GRF WITH FOREFOOT STRIKE
The impact peak is often absent since the collision
force may be a lower magnitude and slightly delayed.
Direction of force increases load on Achilles tendon
and calf and decreases it on tibialis anterior.

COMMON
VARIATIONS

There are several variations seen in natural running gait patterns. Some are due to anatomy, while others come about in response to injury or fatigue. Most gait deviations are not necessarily the cause of injury, and if you display a deviation, it may not make sense to change it. However, if the deviation relates to an injury you've sustained, it may be worth looking into it with a qualified coach or health-care practitioner.

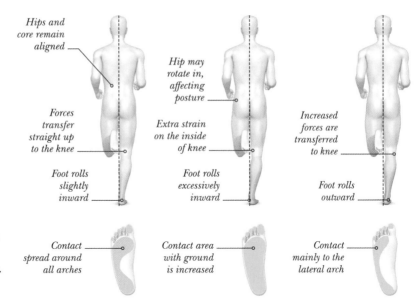

Hips and core remain aligned

Forces transfer straight up to the knee

Foot rolls slightly inward

Contact spread around all arches

Hip may rotate in, affecting posture

Extra strain on the inside of knee

Foot rolls excessively inward

Contact area with ground is increased

Increased forces are transferred to knee

Foot rolls outward

Contact mainly to the lateral arch

Pronation

Pronation is the inward rolling of the foot in the first half of stance phase (see p.67). It is a combined movement that incorporates the ankle, rearfoot, and forefoot joints. Pronation is often portrayed as a bad thing, but it is a necessary and efficient shock-absorption mechanism.

NEUTRAL
Neutral pronation involves landing on the outside of the heel, rolling inward to transfer the force through the midfoot at midstance, and then toeing-off of the end of the big toe.

OVERPRONATION
Excessive pronation tends to cause splaying and transfers force to the inside of the foot. The ankle also tends to rotate in more, which may affect mechanics at the knee and hip.

UNDERPRONATION
Decreased pronation is characterized by a more rigid foot, where the medial arch makes little or no contact with the ground. This results in less shock-absorption capability by the foot.

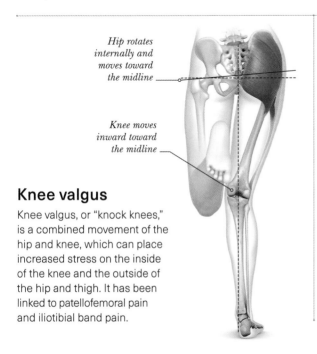

Hip rotates internally and moves toward the midline

Knee moves inward toward the midline

Knee valgus

Knee valgus, or "knock knees," is a combined movement of the hip and knee, which can place increased stress on the inside of the knee and the outside of the hip and thigh. It has been linked to patellofemoral pain and iliotibial band pain.

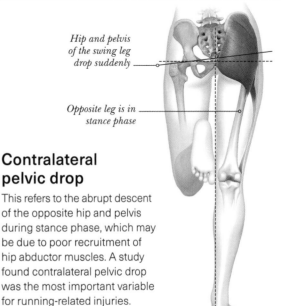

Hip and pelvis of the swing leg drop suddenly

Opposite leg is in stance phase

Contralateral pelvic drop

This refers to the abrupt descent of the opposite hip and pelvis during stance phase, which may be due to poor recruitment of hip abductor muscles. A study found contralateral pelvic drop was the most important variable for running-related injuries.

RUNNING **FORM**

While there is no single ideal running form, coaches and scientists agree there are better ways to run. Keeping in mind your individual biomechanics, by comparing how you run against the form shown here, you might identify ways to streamline your form for greater efficiency and to guard against injury.

POSTURE

Maintaining good posture when running is crucial; it can affect breathing, shock absorption, and power generation. Overall, it is important not to hunch forward and look down at your feet. Instead, imagine a string pulling your head up and extending your spine.

Arms

The arms and shoulders play an important role in keeping your upper body relaxed and in generating power. Your arms work with your legs to drive you forward or up hills and to minimize wasteful lateral (side-to-side) movements.

Core

The core is the body's transition zone between the upper body and lower body. It is the site of many muscle attachments that drive both upper and lower limbs. As such, it needs to be inherently stable in order for these muscles to derive power. To engage the core, imagine your belly button is attached to a string pulling you forward and that your upper body and lower body are rotating counter to each other without inhibiting one another. Practice dissociating these areas in your drills and exercises (see pp.84–89 and 144–155).

Feet

The feet are the interface between your body and the ground, and effective footstrikes can make a big difference to running efficiency. Imagine your feet as springs, absorbing energy on landing and bouncing back to return that energy on toe-off.

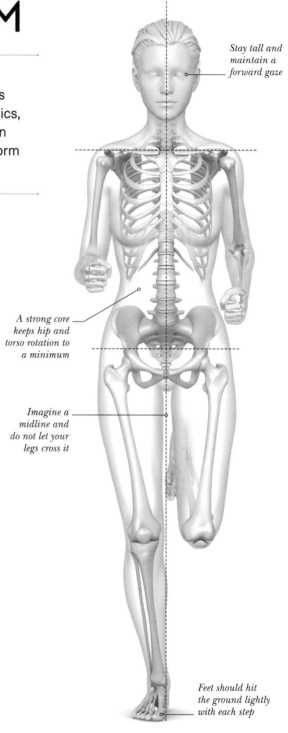

Stay tall and maintain a forward gaze

A strong core keeps hip and torso rotation to a minimum

Imagine a midline and do not let your legs cross it

Feet should hit the ground lightly with each step

ANTERIOR VIEW

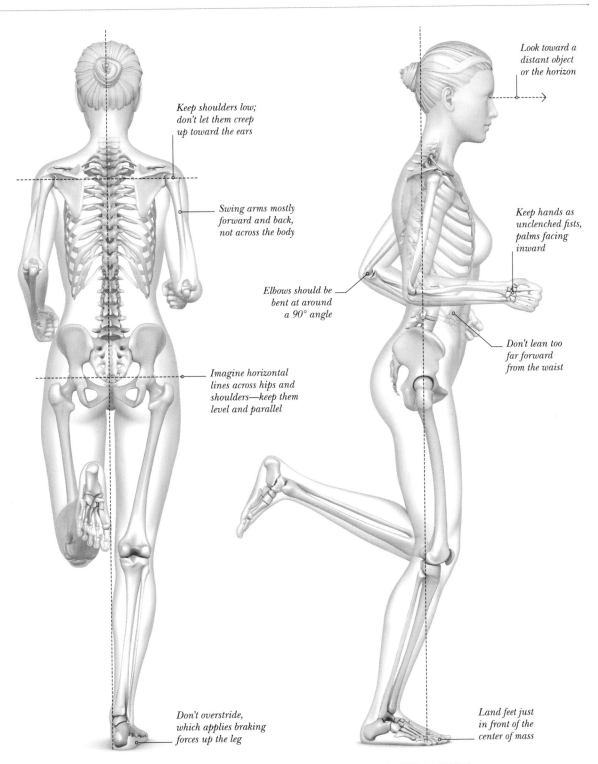

Keep shoulders low;
don't let them creep
up toward the ears

Look toward a
distant object
or the horizon

Swing arms mostly
forward and back,
not across the body

Keep hands as
unclenched fists,
palms facing
inward

Elbows should be
bent at around
a 90° angle

Don't lean too
far forward
from the waist

Imagine horizontal
lines across hips and
shoulders—keep them
level and parallel

Don't overstride,
which applies braking
forces up the leg

Land feet just
in front of the
center of mass

POSTERIOR VIEW

LATERAL VIEW

RUNNING **ROUTINE**

It is sensible to establish warm-up and cool-down routines to bookend your runs. Warming up the body before training with running-specific dynamic stretches and drills enables you to make the most of the workout, while ending it with static stretching helps kick off the recovery process.

50%
REDUCTION IN RISK OF **OVERUSE** **INJURY** IS POSSIBLE FROM A **WARM-UP** PROGRAM

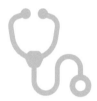

WARM-UP STRETCHES

Dynamic stretches (see pp.78–83) involve movements that take the body through a range of motion, preparing it for activity.

THE BENEFITS

Designed to target the specific movements involved in running, the dynamic stretches in this book increase blood flow to muscles and work on the range of motion of joints. A structured, sport-specific warm-up program can reduce the risk of overuse injuries in running-based sports by up to 50 percent.

HOW TO DO THEM

Start each dynamic stretch with a shallow range of motion at a slow speed, then progress to deeper ranges and greater speeds as your body allows. You should feel that your range of motion increases throughout the stretch. While you are stretching, take the opportunity to assess any asymmetries or restrictions in your movements so you can address them before you begin your workout.

WARM UP AND COOL DOWN

Establish a regular routine for warming up and cooling down around each training session. Ensure you reserve enough time for each stage. Start your workouts with a dynamic warm-up involving stretches and drills, which helps prepare your body for the demands of running, prevents injury, and improves performance. It is especially important on race day that you warm up adequately so you can be confident that you are physically and mentally prepared to do your best. End each run with an adequate cool-down session to begin the recovery process.

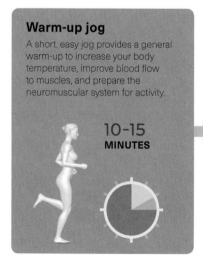

Warm-up jog

A short, easy jog provides a general warm-up to increase your body temperature, improve blood flow to muscles, and prepare the neuromuscular system for activity.

10-15
MINUTES

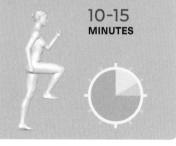

Stretches and drills

A dynamic stretching routine with running-specific drills will take your joints through the required range of motion for running and prepare your neuromuscular system for more intense activity.

10-15
MINUTES

DRILLS

Performing running drills (see pp.84–89) increases blood flow to muscles and the range of motion at your joints. Drills also offer a chance to work on running form and symmetry of movement.

THE BENEFITS

Running drills encourage good form by breaking down running motion into controlled chunks and focusing on specific gait phases.

HOW TO DO THEM

Running drills should be performed 2 or 3 times per week before or after workouts. A good place to carry them out is on a track or field. You need a clear 130–165 ft (40–50 m) to perform the drills. Aim for 15–20 repetitions on each leg.

*Running drills provide an opportunity to work on running **form** and **symmetry** of movement*

RECOVERY STRETCHES

Regular static stretching (see pp.90–95) can help maintain or increase muscle and joint flexibility.

THE BENEFITS

Static stretching is not advised before activity, as it may decrease performance. As part of postrun recovery, it improves joint flexibility and muscle length. While these improvements are not associated with any benefits to performance, stretches can bring helpful relief to tight, hardworking muscles.

HOW TO DO THEM

Static stretches should only be done after exercise. The optimal length of time to hold a static stretch is 30 seconds. Longer holds do not seem to provide additional benefit.

Your run

During your workout, pay attention to your form and any asymmetries or deviations from your normal running gait. As you fatigue, some of these may become more pronounced. Wearable sensors that detect these changes may be useful, as they help you pick up on patterns or changes prior to the onset of pain or injury.

Recovery jog

A slow recovery jog is not really necessary after easy runs but may be beneficial after more intense workouts, enabling you to slow down your heart rate as you gain some extra mileage.

10–15 MINUTES

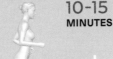

Recovery stretches

Static stretches can encourage you to relax after a hard workout. They may help reduce postrun stiffness and soreness and contribute toward maintaining muscle and joint flexibility.

10 MINUTES

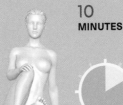

77

Upper body
It is unnecessary to keep your **core** and **pelvis** fixed during the movement. Allow some flexion and extension along the **lumbar spine** to enable a smooth and fluid swinging motion. Also, allow some rotation of the torso, engaging the **obliques** and **pectorals** as your free arm swings forward.

Spine
Spinal extensors
Serratus anterior
Pectoralis major
Rectus abdominis
External oblique

DYNAMIC STRETCH:
FORWARD LEG SWING

This dynamic stretch prepares your body for running by improving flexibility in your hip and posterior leg muscles, which can help prevent injury and improve performance. Use a railing or chair backrest for support. Practice the stretch on each leg in turn, performing 15–20 repetitions or more per side. As you warm up, gradually increase the range of the swinging motion.

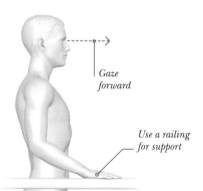

Gaze forward

Use a railing for support

Keep stance leg straight

Soft bend in focus knee

PREPARATORY STAGE
Stand tall, holding onto your support with the arm on the same side of the body as the swinging leg. Shift your weight onto the stance leg, ready to begin the dynamic stretch. Relax the knee of the focus leg to a soft bend.

STAGE ONE
Swing the focus leg forward and reach for your toes with your opposite hand, tapping your toes if possible. Swing your leg like a pendulum, allowing momentum to carry your foot up into the air in front of you and maintaining a soft bend in your knee until you feel a gentle stretch in the back of your thigh, knee, and/or lower leg. Keep the stance knee straight.

KEY

●-- *Joints*

○— *Muscles*

● Shortening under tension

● Lengthening under tension

● Lengthening without tension (stretching)

● Held muscles without motion

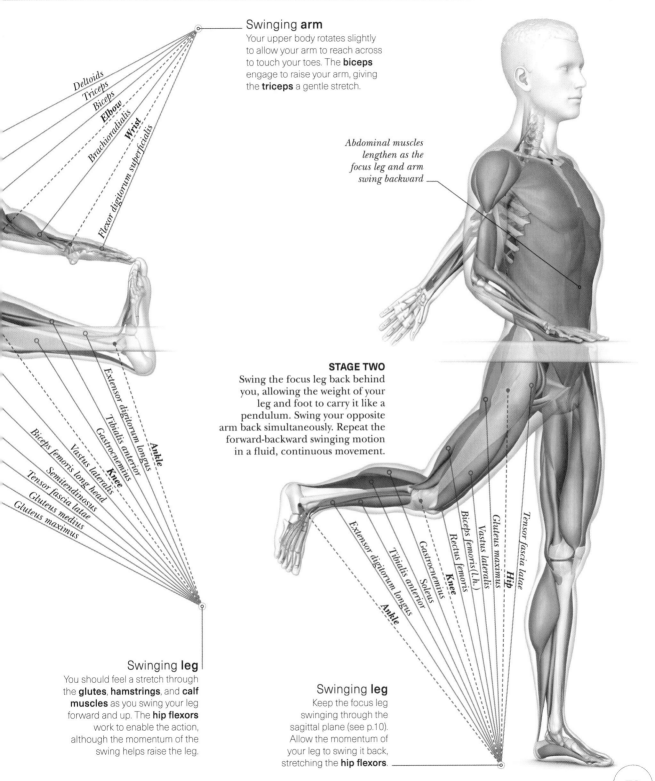

Swinging **arm**

Your upper body rotates slightly to allow your arm to reach across to touch your toes. The **biceps** engage to raise your arm, giving the **triceps** a gentle stretch.

Deltoids
Triceps
Biceps
Elbow
Brachioradialis
Wrist
Flexor digitorum superficialis

Abdominal muscles lengthen as the focus leg and arm swing backward

Extensor digitorum longus
Tibialis anterior
Gastrocnemius
Knee
Vastus lateralis
Biceps femoris long head
Semitendinosus
Tensor fascia latae
Gluteus medius
Gluteus maximus
Ankle

STAGE TWO

Swing the focus leg back behind you, allowing the weight of your leg and foot to carry it like a pendulum. Swing your opposite arm back simultaneously. Repeat the forward-backward swinging motion in a fluid, continuous movement.

Tensor fascia latae
Hip
Gluteus maximus
Vastus lateralis
Biceps femoris (l.h.)
Rectus femoris
Knee
Gastrocnemius
Soleus
Tibialis anterior
Extensor digitorum longus
Ankle

Swinging **leg**

You should feel a stretch through the **glutes**, **hamstrings**, and **calf muscles** as you swing your leg forward and up. The **hip flexors** work to enable the action, although the momentum of the swing helps raise the leg.

Swinging **leg**

Keep the focus leg swinging through the sagittal plane (see p.10). Allow the momentum of your leg to swing it back, stretching the **hip flexors**.

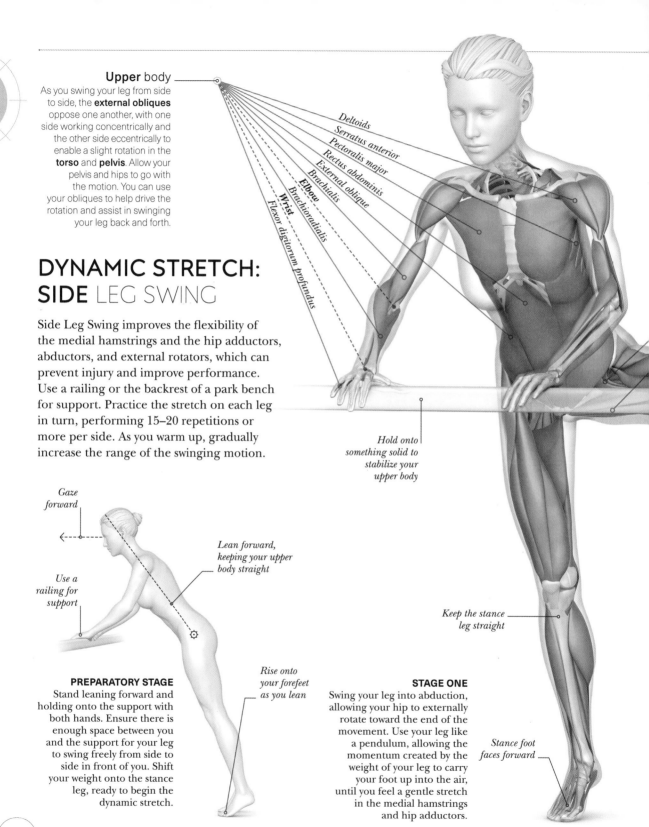

Upper body

As you swing your leg from side to side, the **external obliques** oppose one another, with one side working concentrically and the other side eccentrically to enable a slight rotation in the **torso** and **pelvis**. Allow your pelvis and hips to go with the motion. You can use your obliques to help drive the rotation and assist in swinging your leg back and forth.

Deltoids
Serratus anterior
Pectoralis major
Rectus abdominis
External oblique
Elbow
Brachialis
Wrist
Brachioradialis
Flexor digitorum profundus

DYNAMIC STRETCH: SIDE LEG SWING

Side Leg Swing improves the flexibility of the medial hamstrings and the hip adductors, abductors, and external rotators, which can prevent injury and improve performance. Use a railing or the backrest of a park bench for support. Practice the stretch on each leg in turn, performing 15–20 repetitions or more per side. As you warm up, gradually increase the range of the swinging motion.

Hold onto something solid to stabilize your upper body

Gaze forward

Lean forward, keeping your upper body straight

Use a railing for support

Keep the stance leg straight

PREPARATORY STAGE
Stand leaning forward and holding onto the support with both hands. Ensure there is enough space between you and the support for your leg to swing freely from side to side in front of you. Shift your weight onto the stance leg, ready to begin the dynamic stretch.

Rise onto your forefeet as you lean

STAGE ONE
Swing your leg into abduction, allowing your hip to externally rotate toward the end of the movement. Use your leg like a pendulum, allowing the momentum created by the weight of your leg to carry your foot up into the air, until you feel a gentle stretch in the medial hamstrings and hip adductors.

Stance foot faces forward

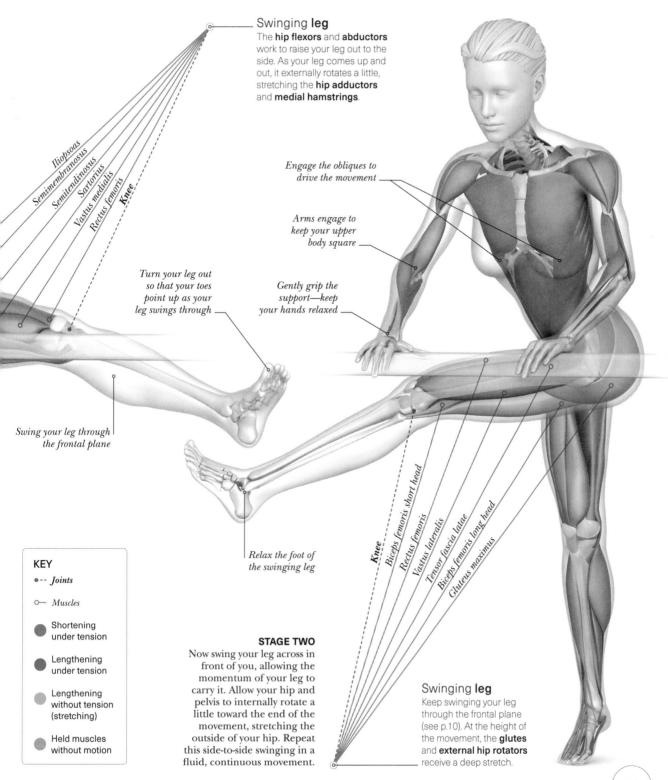

Swinging leg
The **hip flexors** and **abductors** work to raise your leg out to the side. As your leg comes up and out, it externally rotates a little, stretching the **hip adductors** and **medial hamstrings**.

Iliopsoas

Semimembranosus

Semitendinosus

Sartorius

Vastus medialis

Rectus femoris

Knee

Engage the obliques to drive the movement

Arms engage to keep your upper body square

Turn your leg out so that your toes point up as your leg swings through

Gently grip the support—keep your hands relaxed

Swing your leg through the frontal plane

Relax the foot of the swinging leg

Knee

Biceps femoris short head

Rectus femoris

Vastus lateralis

Tensor fascia latae

Biceps femoris long head

Gluteus maximus

KEY

●-- *Joints*

○— *Muscles*

● Shortening under tension

● Lengthening under tension

● Lengthening without tension (stretching)

● Held muscles without motion

STAGE TWO
Now swing your leg across in front of you, allowing the momentum of your leg to carry it. Allow your hip and pelvis to internally rotate a little toward the end of the movement, stretching the outside of your hip. Repeat this side-to-side swinging in a fluid, continuous movement.

Swinging leg
Keep swinging your leg through the frontal plane (see p.10). At the height of the movement, the **glutes** and **external hip rotators** receive a deep stretch.

81

DYNAMIC STRETCH: CALF STRETCH

This stretch improves the flexibility of your calf and Achilles tendon, helping prevent injury and improve performance. Lean on a wall or railing for support during the exercise. Perform 15–20 repetitions or more, gradually pushing your heel down further as you warm up. Do not hold the stretch, but move fluidly between the stages in a continuous repetitive flow. The variation (opposite) stretches the soleus muscle rather than the gastrocnemius.

KEY

- •-- *Joints*
- o— *Muscles*
- ● Shortening under tension
- ● Lengthening under tension
- ● Lengthening without tension (stretching)
- ● Held muscles without motion

PREPARATORY STAGE
Rest your hands on the support, then step back to increase the angle of your lean to roughly 45°, with your body forming a straight line from your heels to the top of your head. Your heels should be just off the ground and your knees should be slightly soft.

Gaze forward

Lean on a stable support

Lean forward

Soft bend in the knees

Feet are together, heels slightly raised

Upper **body**
Lean your weight into the railing to support your upper body. Your **arm**, **upper torso**, and **core muscles** engage to hold your upper body straight.

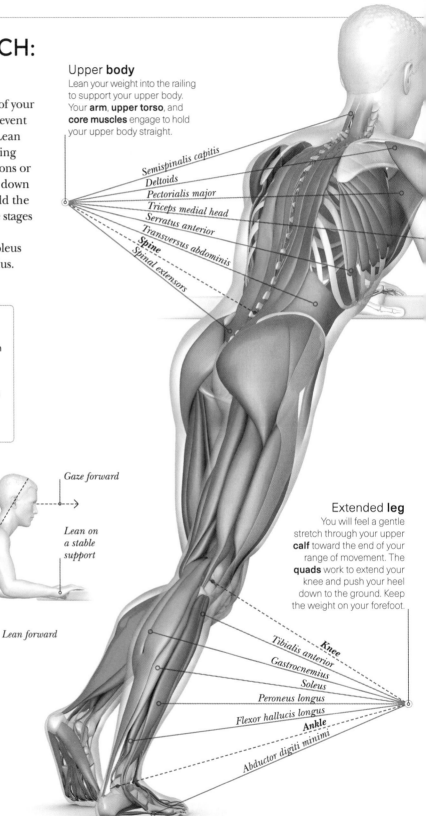

Semispinalis capitis
Deltoids
Pectoralis major
Triceps medial head
Serratus anterior
Transversus abdominis
Spine
Spinal extensors

Extended **leg**
You will feel a gentle stretch through your upper **calf** toward the end of your range of movement. The **quads** work to extend your knee and push your heel down to the ground. Keep the weight on your forefoot.

Knee
Tibialis anterior
Gastrocnemius
Soleus
Peroneus longus
Flexor hallucis longus
Ankle
Abductor digiti minimi

STAGE ONE
Bend your left knee and raise
your left heel off the ground
to bring the weight onto your
forefoot. Simultaneously, push
down toward the floor with
your right heel and extend
your right knee. You should
feel a gentle stretch in your
right upper calf. As soon as
you feel the stretch, move
fluidly into stage 2.

STAGE TWO
Reverse the movement.
Unlock the right knee and
raise the right heel off the
floor while you push down
with your left heel and extend
your left knee. Repeat stages
1 and 2 in a continuous
movement.

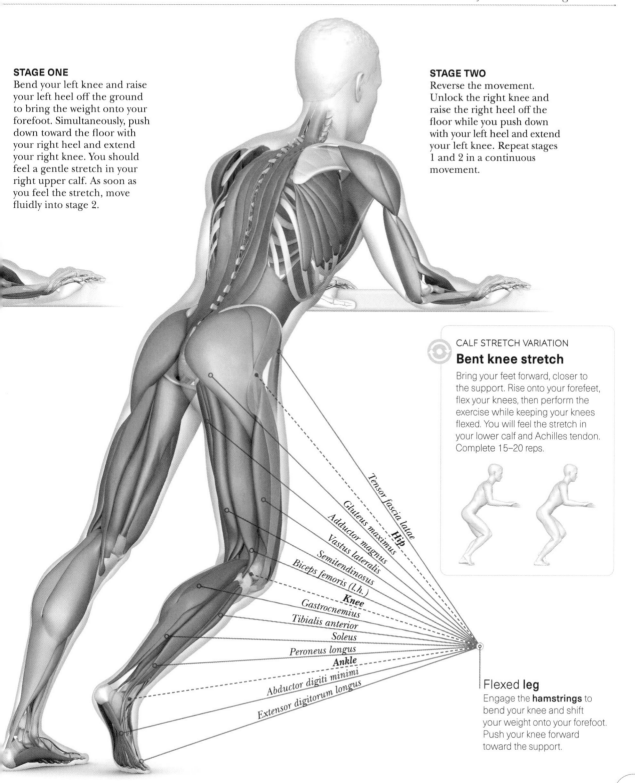

CALF STRETCH VARIATION
Bent knee stretch

Bring your feet forward, closer to
the support. Rise onto your forefeet,
flex your knees, then perform the
exercise while keeping your knees
flexed. You will feel the stretch in
your lower calf and Achilles tendon.
Complete 15–20 reps.

Tensor fascia latae
Hip
Gluteus maximus
Adductor magnus
Vastus lateralis
Semitendinosus
Biceps femoris (l.h.)
Knee
Gastrocnemius
Tibialis anterior
Soleus
Peroneus longus
Ankle
Abductor digiti minimi
Extensor digitorum longus

Flexed **leg**
Engage the **hamstrings** to
bend your knee and shift
your weight onto your forefoot.
Push your knee forward
toward the support.

DRILLS: RUNNING As

This marching drill emphasizes a driving knee lift, coordinated arm and leg movements, and good posture by maintaining a slight forward lean in the body. Your muscles must work hard to achieve the high-knee motion, which warms up the body and helps it tune in to good running form. Try to keep light on your feet and note that the steps, while exaggerated, are small, allowing for a slow progression forward.

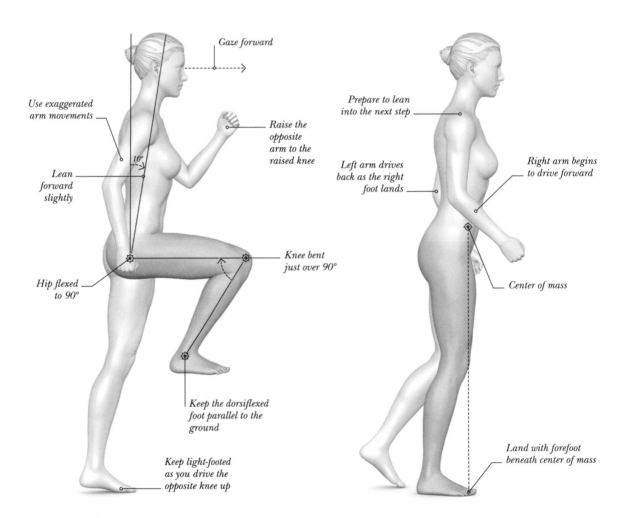

Gaze forward

Use exaggerated arm movements

Raise the opposite arm to the raised knee

Lean forward slightly

10°

Hip flexed to 90°

Knee bent just over 90°

Keep the dorsiflexed foot parallel to the ground

Keep light-footed as you drive the opposite knee up

Prepare to lean into the next step

Right arm begins to drive forward

Left arm drives back as the right foot lands

Center of mass

Land with forefoot beneath center of mass

DRIVE THE KNEE UP
Stand tall, leaning forward slightly. Raise the right knee high and swing your arms in running motion. As you drive into the next step, allow the left heel to raise off the ground so your weight rests on the forefoot.

TAKE SMALL STEPS
Quickly return the right leg to the ground slightly ahead of the opposite foot, landing on the forefoot. Drive the opposite arm back in running motion. Repeat for 15–20 repetitions per leg.

DRILLS: RUNNING Bs

Adding a swift knee extension after driving the knee up
challenges the hamstrings in this drill. The quick movement
makes the sequence feel similar to skipping. Try to make the
movements as smooth and fluid as possible. Regular practice
improves stability in the lower limbs and increases the range
of motion available in the hip, knee, and ankle joints.

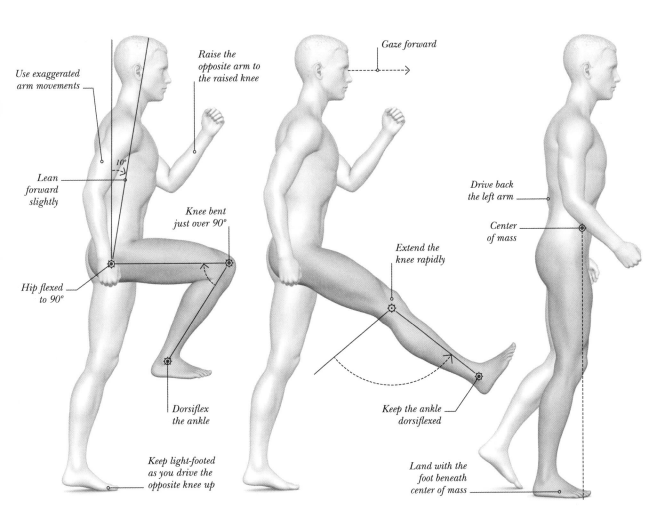

Use exaggerated arm movements

Raise the opposite arm to the raised knee

10°

Lean forward slightly

Knee bent just over 90°

Hip flexed to 90°

Dorsiflex the ankle

Keep light-footed as you drive the opposite knee up

Gaze forward

Extend the knee rapidly

Keep the ankle dorsiflexed

Drive back the left arm

Center of mass

Land with the foot beneath center of mass

DRIVE THE KNEE UP
Stand tall, leaning forward slightly.
Raise the right knee high and swing
your arms in running motion. As
you drive forward into the next
step, allow the left heel to raise
off the ground.

EXTEND THE KNEE
Just as you begin to pull the
leg back down to the ground,
extend the knee powerfully to
straighten the leg.

LAND UNDER CENTER OF MASS
Swiftly sweep the extended leg back
underneath you and land the right
foot slightly ahead of the left, with
the forefoot beneath your center
of mass. Drive the left arm back
in running motion.

DRILLS: RUNNING Cs

This drill incorporates a butt kick with each stride as you drive
forward smoothly in small, positive running steps. Regular
practice promotes hip flexor and quadriceps flexibility, as well
as efficient footwork and running cadence. Move the arms in a
running motion, raising the opposite arm to the raised leg, or
if you find this distracting, hold them by your waist and focus
your attention on the movement.

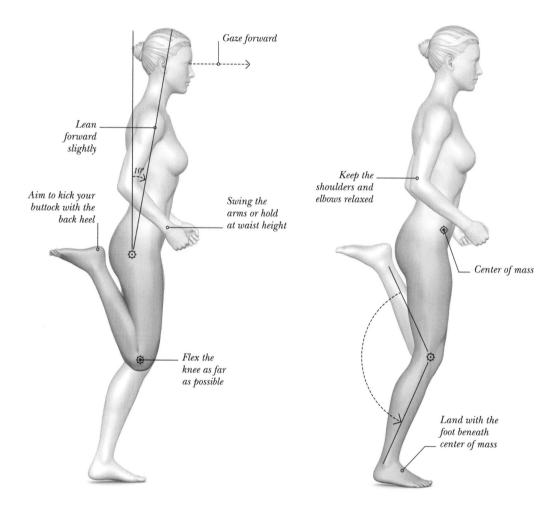

Gaze forward

*Lean
forward
slightly*

10°

*Aim to kick your
buttock with the
back heel*

*Swing the
arms or hold
at waist height*

*Flex the
knee as far
as possible*

*Keep the
shoulders and
elbows relaxed*

Center of mass

*Land with the
foot beneath
center of mass*

KICK ONE SIDE
Stand tall with a slight forward lean.
Snap your right heel up toward your
buttock, keeping the left leg straight
as you drive into the next step. Allow
the left heel to raise off the ground
so your weight rests on the forefoot.

KICK THE OPPOSITE SIDE
Immediately bring the right leg back
to the ground after a short flight phase
(when both feet are off the ground).
Land with the forefoot beneath your
center of mass and slightly ahead of
the opposite foot.

DRILLS: STRIDES

Strides allow you to perfect your form at speed. Make your strides a slightly exaggerated version of your running form. Begin at a comfortable pace, focusing on posture and footwork, then accelerate during the set to roughly 80 percent of your maximum speed for the final 5–10 seconds.

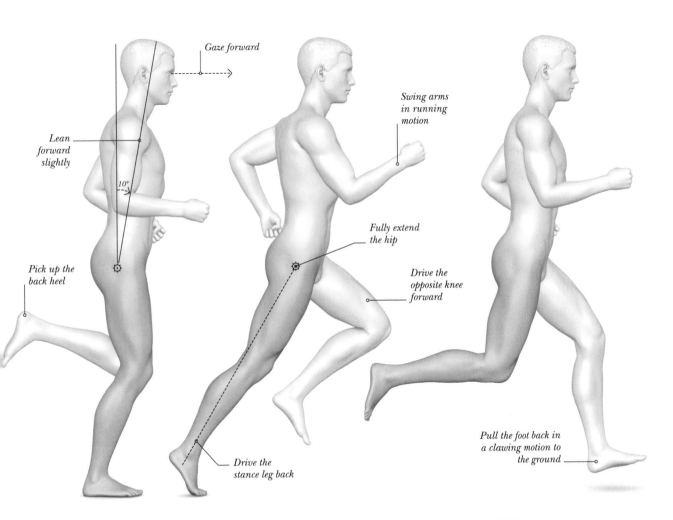

Gaze forward

Lean forward slightly

10°

Pick up the back heel

Swing arms in running motion

Fully extend the hip

Drive the opposite knee forward

Drive the stance leg back

Pull the foot back in a clawing motion to the ground

FOCUS ON FORM
Stand tall with a slight forward lean as you begin your set of strides. Focus on your form, ensuring your forefoot or heel (whichever is natural to you) lands beneath your hips. Keep your shoulders relaxed.

PICK UP SPEED
As you accelerate, ensure that you drive the stance leg back and pull the opposite knee up and forward with each step. A strong knee drive creates a powerful hip extension in the stance leg for push-off.

FINAL SPRINT
Maintain your form as you power into a sprint at 80 percent of your maximum speed for a short burst to end the set. Drive your arms back and forth in running motion as you run to help power your movement.

DRILLS: BOUNDING

The bounding drill increases the power of your leg springs.
As you land, aim to drive straight through into an explosive
take-off, then continue powerfully with the opposite knee. Aim
to bound as high and as far forward as you can, then hold the
sprint position at the height of the movement briefly before
landing with some velocity, ready to spring forward again.

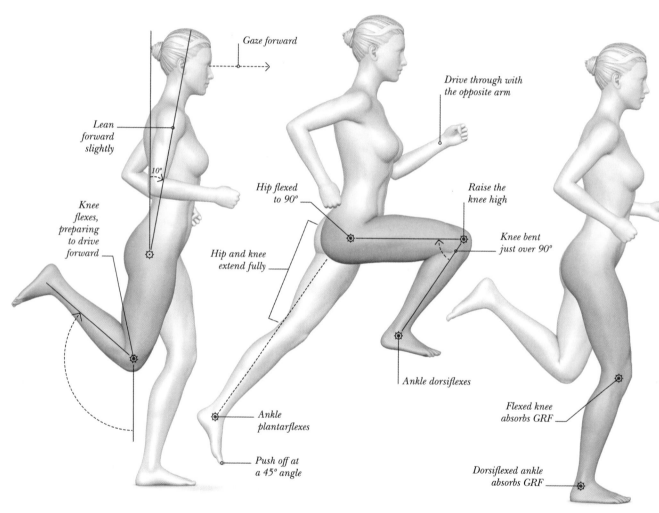

Gaze forward

*Drive through with
the opposite arm*

*Lean
forward
slightly*

10°

*Hip flexed
to 90°*

*Raise the
knee high*

*Knee
flexes,
preparing
to drive
forward*

*Hip and knee
extend fully*

*Knee bent
just over 90°*

Ankle dorsiflexes

*Ankle
plantarflexes*

*Flexed knee
absorbs GRF*

*Push off at
a 45° angle*

*Dorsiflexed ankle
absorbs GRF*

PREPARE TO DRIVE THE KNEE
As you land, lean forward from
the ankle with your weight on
the forefoot and with your knee
and hip slightly flexed. Flex the
opposite knee, ready to drive it
up with the next stride.

PUSH OFF EXPLOSIVELY
Push off strongly in an exaggerated
running motion to drive yourself up
and forward off the ground. Drive
the opposite knee forward and the
arms through in running motion to
help propel you off the ground.

LAND SOFTLY
As you land and start absorbing the
ground reaction force (GRF), focus
on powering through into the next
stride. Think of your leg as a spring,
storing GRF energy to propel
explosively forward and upward.

DRILLS: CARIOCA

The carioca drill is a sideways movement that helps improve a runner's agility, coordination, and mobility. Aim to make the movements quick and fluid. As the drill becomes familiar, increase your speed to keep the coordinated movement challenging. Move first in one direction, then immediately travel back in the opposite direction to complete a set.

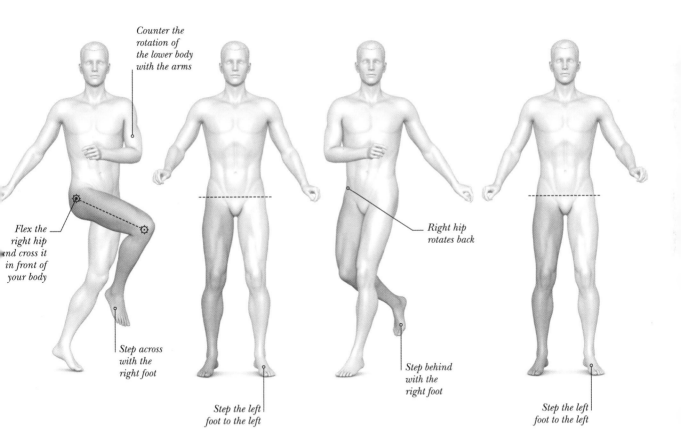

Counter the rotation of the lower body with the arms

Flex the right hip and cross it in front of your body

Step across with the right foot

Step the left foot to the left

Right hip rotates back

Step behind with the right foot

Step the left foot to the left

STEP ACROSS THE FRONT
Start slightly raised on your forefeet. To travel to your left, focus on your right leg. Raise your right knee and step across your body to the left.

STEP TO THE SIDE
Step your left foot out to the left. Remain springy and light-footed on your forefeet.

STEP ACROSS THE BACK
Now pull your right hip back and cross your right leg back and behind your left.

STEP TO THE SIDE
Step your left foot to the left. To travel to your right, focus on your left leg and reverse the directions.

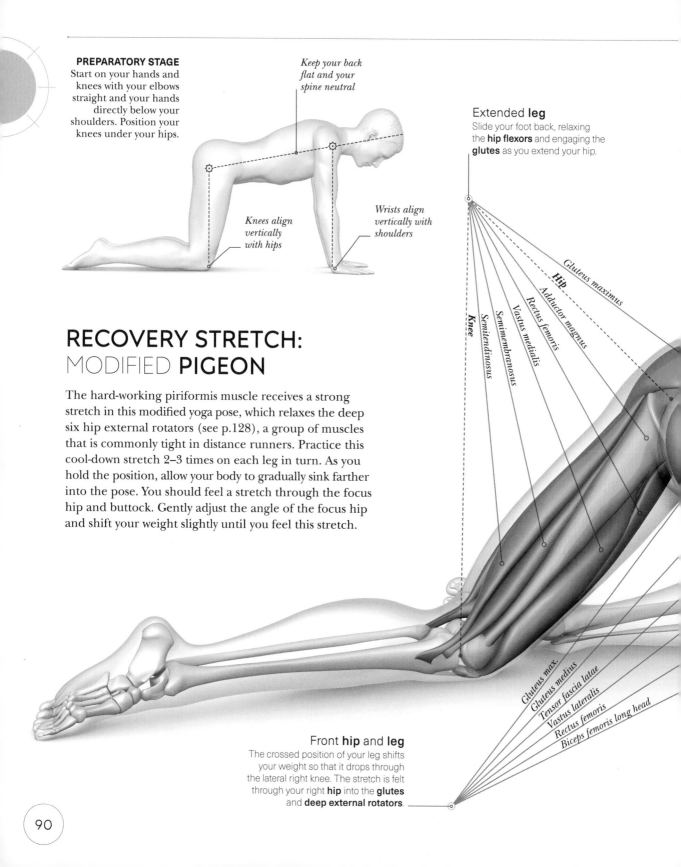

PREPARATORY STAGE
Start on your hands and
knees with your elbows
straight and your hands
directly below your
shoulders. Position your
knees under your hips.

*Keep your back
flat and your
spine neutral*

*Knees align
vertically
with hips*

*Wrists align
vertically with
shoulders*

Extended **leg**
Slide your foot back, relaxing
the **hip flexors** and engaging the
glutes as you extend your hip.

Gluteus maximus
Hip
Adductor magnus
Rectus femoris
Vastus medialis
Semimembranosus
Semitendinosus
Knee

RECOVERY STRETCH:
MODIFIED **PIGEON**

The hard-working piriformis muscle receives a strong
stretch in this modified yoga pose, which relaxes the deep
six hip external rotators (see p.128), a group of muscles
that is commonly tight in distance runners. Practice this
cool-down stretch 2–3 times on each leg in turn. As you
hold the position, allow your body to gradually sink farther
into the pose. You should feel a stretch through the focus
hip and buttock. Gently adjust the angle of the focus hip
and shift your weight slightly until you feel this stretch.

Gluteus max.
Gluteus medius
Tensor fascia latae
Vastus lateralis
Rectus femoris
Biceps femoris long head

Front **hip** and **leg**
The crossed position of your leg shifts
your weight so that it drops through
the lateral right knee. The stretch is felt
through your right **hip** into the **glutes**
and **deep external rotators**.

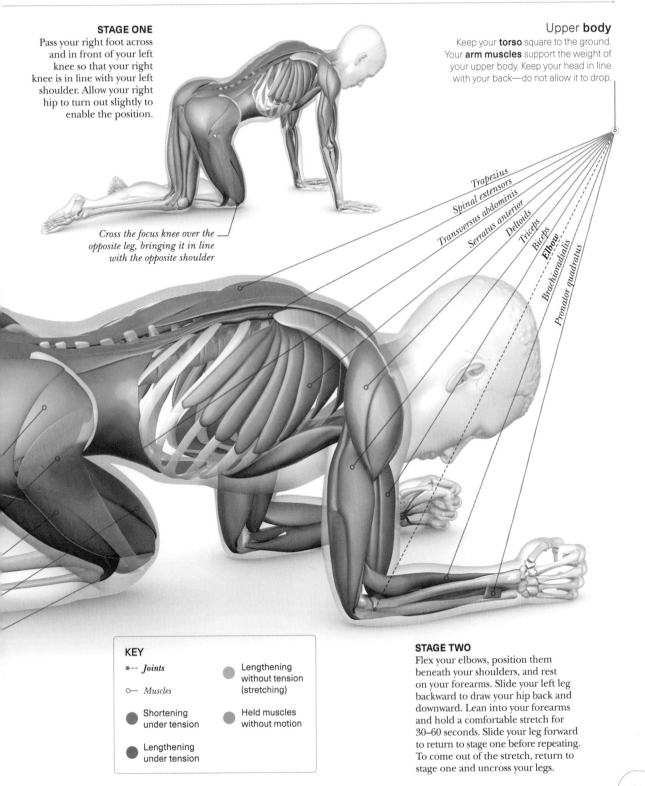

STAGE ONE
Pass your right foot across and in front of your left knee so that your right knee is in line with your left shoulder. Allow your right hip to turn out slightly to enable the position.

Cross the focus knee over the opposite leg, bringing it in line with the opposite shoulder

Upper **body**
Keep your **torso** square to the ground. Your **arm muscles** support the weight of your upper body. Keep your head in line with your back—do not allow it to drop.

Trapezius
Spinal extensors
Transversus abdominis
Serratus anterior
Deltoids
Triceps
Biceps
Elbow
Brachioradialis
Pronator quadratus

KEY

- •-- *Joints*
- ○— *Muscles*
- ● Shortening under tension
- ● Lengthening under tension
- ● Lengthening without tension (stretching)
- ● Held muscles without motion

STAGE TWO
Flex your elbows, position them beneath your shoulders, and rest on your forearms. Slide your left leg backward to draw your hip back and downward. Lean into your forearms and hold a comfortable stretch for 30–60 seconds. Slide your leg forward to return to stage one before repeating. To come out of the stretch, return to stage one and uncross your legs.

91

RECOVERY STRETCH:
TFL BALL RELEASE

If you have recently increased your training load, or if your occupation requires you to sit for prolonged periods, you might find your tensor fascia latae (TFL) muscles are frequently tight. This active-release exercise using a ball relaxes the TFL. Select a harder lacrosse-style therapy ball rather than a soft foam one. Start by applying light pressure on the ball, increasing this gradually as your body allows. Repeat 10–12 times on each side, or for as long as needed, to feel a release in the TFL muscle.

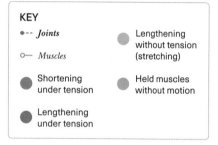

KEY

•-- *Joints*

o— *Muscles*

● Shortening under tension

● Lengthening under tension

● Lengthening without tension (stretching)

● Held muscles without motion

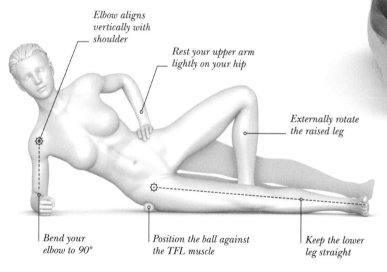

Elbow aligns vertically with shoulder

Rest your upper arm lightly on your hip

Externally rotate the raised leg

Bend your elbow to 90°

Position the ball against the TFL muscle

Keep the lower leg straight

STAGE ONE
Using the raised leg to control the amount of weight you apply to the ball, allow the weight of your hip to gradually sink down onto the ball. Once comfortable with the pressure on the TFL, flex the hip and knee of the lower leg to approximately 30° while keeping the ball in place under the TFL. You should feel a strong sensation across the TFL and possibly in the buttock, lateral thigh, and groin areas.

PREPARATORY STAGE
Lie down on one side with your legs straight. Prop yourself up on one arm. Flex the upper knee, raise the leg, and bring the heel to the floor behind the straight knee. Press into the foot to raise your hip off the floor and place the ball between the floor and the center of the TFL muscle. Gently roll your torso forward slightly if necessary to hold the ball in place.

Lower **hip**
The **hip flexors** engage to bend your hip, while the **TFL** receives an intense stretch. The **hamstrings** engage to bend the knee as you raise it toward your chest.

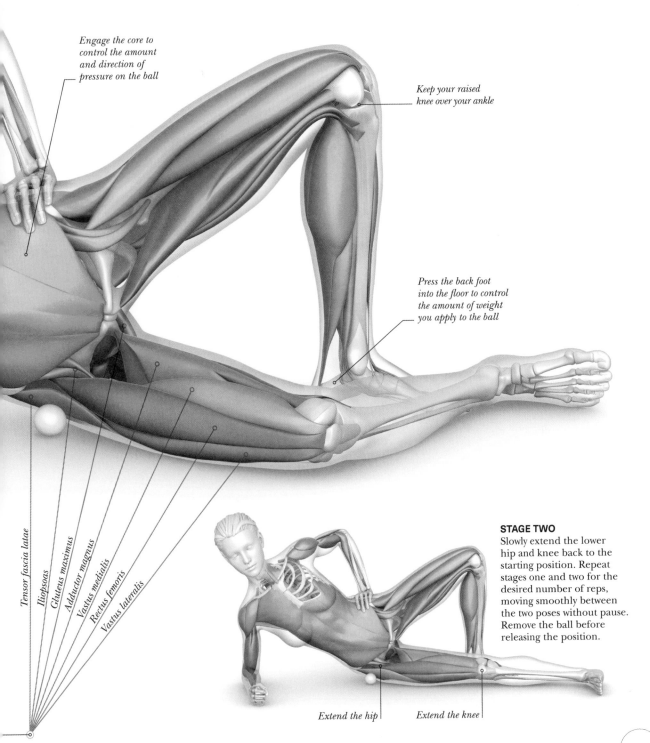

Engage the core to
control the amount
and direction of
pressure on the ball

Keep your raised
knee over your ankle

Press the back foot
into the floor to control
the amount of weight
you apply to the ball

Tensor fascia latae
Iliopsoas
Gluteus maximus
Adductor magnus
Vastus medialis
Rectus femoris
Vastus lateralis

STAGE TWO

Slowly extend the lower
hip and knee back to the
starting position. Repeat
stages one and two for the
desired number of reps,
moving smoothly between
the two poses without pause.
Remove the ball before
releasing the position.

Extend the hip

Extend the knee

RECOVERY STRETCH:
PIRIFORMIS BALL RELEASE

This active-release exercise using a therapy ball (see p.92) relaxes the piriformis muscle, which can become tight with increased training volume and sedentary occupations. Start by applying your weight lightly on the ball as you move your knee from side to side in a fluid, continuous movement. Increase the amount of pressure gradually, as your body allows. Repeat 10–12 times on each leg, or for as long as needed, to feel a release in the piriformis.

Upper **body**
The **deltoids** and **triceps** in the supporting arm engage to prop up your upper body, while the muscles of the active arm guide the rotational movement of your hip via your knee.

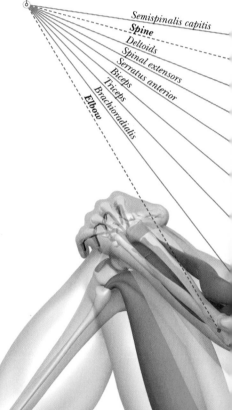

Semispinalis capitis
Spine
Deltoids
Spinal extensors
Serratus anterior
Biceps
Triceps
Brachioradialis
Elbow

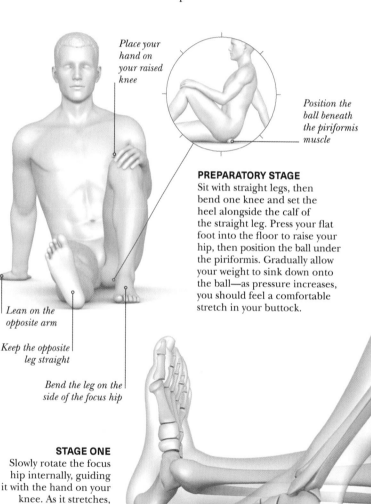

Place your hand on your raised knee

Position the ball beneath the piriformis muscle

PREPARATORY STAGE
Sit with straight legs, then bend one knee and set the heel alongside the calf of the straight leg. Press your flat foot into the floor to raise your hip, then position the ball under the piriformis. Gradually allow your weight to sink down onto the ball—as pressure increases, you should feel a comfortable stretch in your buttock.

Lean on the opposite arm

Keep the opposite leg straight

Bend the leg on the side of the focus hip

STAGE ONE
Slowly rotate the focus hip internally, guiding it with the hand on your knee. As it stretches, you will feel a strong sensation across the piriformis and possibly in your thigh, groin, or buttock.

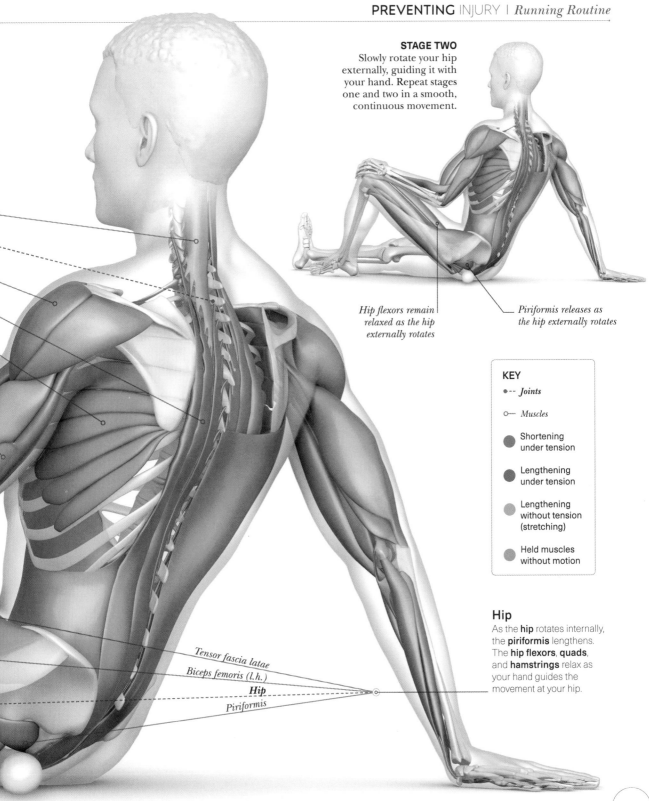

STAGE TWO
Slowly rotate your hip externally, guiding it with your hand. Repeat stages one and two in a smooth, continuous movement.

Hip flexors remain relaxed as the hip externally rotates

Piriformis releases as the hip externally rotates

KEY

●-- *Joints*

○— *Muscles*

● Shortening under tension

● Lengthening under tension

● Lengthening without tension (stretching)

● Held muscles without motion

Hip

As the **hip** rotates internally, the **piriformis** lengthens. The **hip flexors**, **quads**, and **hamstrings** relax as your hand guides the movement at your hip.

Tensor fascia latae
Biceps femoris (l.h.)
Hip
Piriformis

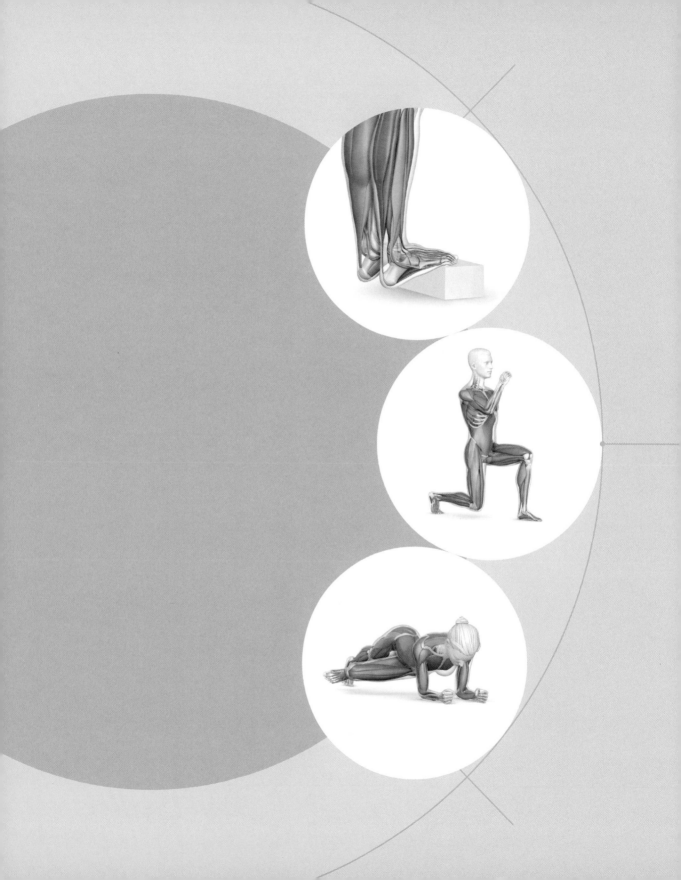

STRENGTH
EXERCISES

Selected for their focus on the muscles used most in running,
the strength-training exercises featured in this chapter can be used to
develop the power and robustness needed to withstand the repetitive
impacts involved in running, as well as the increasing loads of a training
program. There is growing evidence to suggest that strength training
has a beneficial effect not only on injury risk, but also on performance.

PLANNING YOUR DRILLS

Regular strength training using the exercises in this chapter can complement your running and become a valuable cross-training activity (see p.187). By understanding which muscles are working, the joint actions involved, and how each drill benefits your training, you can ensure you are exercising optimally and gaining the maximum benefit.

WHY DO STRENGTH TRAINING?

If fast, pain-free running is your goal, it may seem counterintuitive to do any training other than running. However, the reality is that strength training can improve running performance and economy and reduce the risk of injury.

TARGETED TRAINING

The storage and release of energy in your tendons (see pp.18–19) contributes up to half of the total work involved in each step. Targeting the efficiency of this process can have significant effects on running performance. Increasing the "stiffness" of the tendons is one way to do this. Stiffness, in the biomechanical sense, is the extent to which a structure resists deformation in response to an externally applied force. Stiffer tendons can store more energy when stretched in the loading phase of running and release more energy during the propulsion phase.

IMPROVING STIFFNESS

Increasing the stiffness of tendons requires high loads and greater time under tension. Running can produce loads of up to only 2.5–3 times' body weight and places tendons under tension for short periods of time (when your foot is in contact with the ground).

Heavy resistance training offers an opportunity to increase tendon stiffness under loads greater than those achieved during running and for longer periods, thereby improving running performance.

> **! Caution**
> Pay attention to cautions indicated alongside exercise instructions. If you find you experience pain while practicing any exercise, consult a physical therapist to establish the cause and avoid aggravating an existing condition. If you experience pain greater than 3/10 (see p.56), discontinue the exercise until you are advised otherwise by your clinician.

Enhancing impact absorption and propulsion

Some of the exercises in this chapter increase the capacity of the lower limbs (see p.18) to absorb the ground reaction force (GRF). Others improve the body's ability to generate propulsive power (see p.19). Several of the exercises provide both benefits. Ensure you include a combination of these exercises in your regular drills.

Exercises that improve propulsion capacity

- Hip Extension
- Step Up
- Hamstring Ball Roll-in

- Lunge
- Box Jump
- Single Leg Hop
- Heel Drop
- Traditional Deadlift
- Romanian deadlift
- Single Leg Ball Squat

Exercises that improve GRF absorption capacity

- Hip Hike
- Step Down

PERFORMING **THE EXERCISES**

Most of the 18 exercises and variations in this chapter involve repeated movements between two poses, either held for a specific length of time or continued fluidly between poses. Pay attention to timings and covering the complete range of movement for each exercise, following all of the form and alignment tips.

For each exercise, the main image features the movement that is the main focus. To ensure you work each side of the body in isolation, there is often a target or focus leg and a nonfocus leg. This is important, since in running you are only ever on one leg at a time. Progressions for exercises are provided where they exist; otherwise, when you find you are no longer working hard, move on

to a more difficult version of the exercise. Often, progressions add the use of weights (see right), but sometimes you will move on to a different exercise altogether.

ESTABLISHING A REGIMEN

If you are just starting out and have no injuries, choose 3–5 exercises that target the hip, thigh, and calf muscles. Aim for 2 sessions per week for at least 6 weeks in order to see strength gains. Perform the stated number of reps and sets on each side of the body (alternating sides between sets), ensuring there is enough resistance for your muscles to feel fatigued by the end of each set. Take 2–3 minutes recovery time between sets. If you are rehabilitating a specific injury, follow the guidance of your physical therapist.

What you will need

While most of the exercises do not involve the use of props, you will need to invest in a few pieces of equipment if you lack access to a gym:

- Resistance bands—use bands of increasing strengths as you become stronger
- Exercise step/box—high (12 in/ 30 cm) and low (6 in/15 cm)
- Exercise mat for floor exercises, if desired
- Barbell for deadlifts
- Dumbbells of various weights— switch to heavier weights as you become stronger
- Backpack for weights (see below)
- Exercise ball—21½ in (55 cm) or 26 in (65 cm) diameter

Many of the exercises instruct you to "add weight" once an exercise becomes easy. You can simply perform the exercise holding dumbbells, if the body position will allow it. Alternatively, wear a backpack containing weights, adding more as required to progress.

Injury prevention and rehabilitations

Many of the exercises in this book can be used to help you rehabilitate from a number of common running-related injuries. Those exercises also help protect

against the same injuries. If you are prone to or rehabilitating from any of the injuries below, focus on the listed exercises.

IT band pain (see p.61)
- Hip Hike
- Standing Hip Rotation
- Single Leg Ball Squat
- Step Down
- Step Up
- Hip Extension
- Lunge
- Box Jump (advanced)

Patellofemoral pain (see p.57)
- Hip Hike
- Standing Hip Rotation
- Step Down
- Step Up
- Single Leg Ball Squat
- Traditional Deadlift
- Lunge
- Box Jump (advanced)
- Single Leg Hop

Ankle sprains and chronic ankle instability
- Ankle Eversion
- Ankle Inversion
- Resisted Toe
- Foot Doming
- Single Leg Hop

Achilles tendinopathy (see p.58)
- Heel Drop, including seated variation
- Dynamic Calf Stretch
- Single Leg Hop (advanced)

Hamstring tendinopathy
- Hamstring Ball Roll In
- Hip Extension
- Traditional Deadlift
- Romanian Deadlift

Plantar heel pain (see p.60)
- Resisted Toe
- Foot Doming
- Ankle Turn In
- Single Leg Hop (advanced)

FOOT DOMING

This exercise targets the intrinsic muscles of the foot (see p.102), enhancing the foot's springlike nature to aid in performance. Regular practice improves the function and stability of the foot and ankle, which may benefit runners with chronic ankle instability from repeated sprains.

THE BIG PICTURE

The foot core (see p.22) is your target in this exercise. During stage one, you raise it in a dome shape, decreasing the distance between the heel and the first big toe joint.

If new to this exercise, perform 3–4 sets of 10–12 reps. To advance, work through the following progressions, performing the exercise: while standing; while standing on one leg; while holding a squat; while holding a single-leg squat; holding stage one while stepping forward; holding stage one while stepping onto, then down from, a step; and holding stage one while hopping.

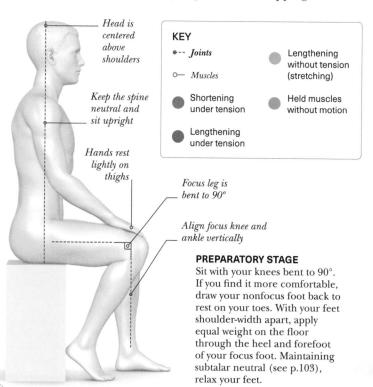

Head is centered above shoulders

Keep the spine neutral and sit upright

Hands rest lightly on thighs

Focus leg is bent to 90°

Align focus knee and ankle vertically

KEY

- - - *Joints*

○— *Muscles*

● Shortening under tension

● Lengthening under tension

● Lengthening without tension (stretching)

● Held muscles without motion

PREPARATORY STAGE
Sit with your knees bent to 90°. If you find it more comfortable, draw your nonfocus foot back to rest on your toes. With your feet shoulder-width apart, apply equal weight on the floor through the heel and forefoot of your focus foot. Maintaining subtalar neutral (see p.103), relax your feet.

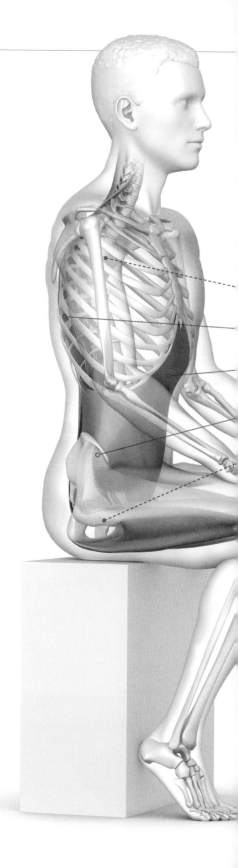

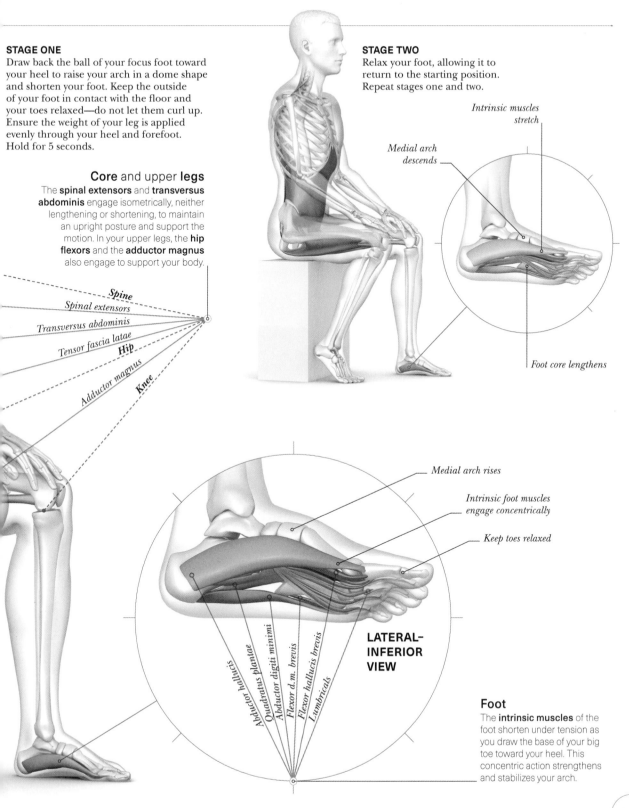

STAGE ONE

Draw back the ball of your focus foot toward your heel to raise your arch in a dome shape and shorten your foot. Keep the outside of your foot in contact with the floor and your toes relaxed—do not let them curl up. Ensure the weight of your leg is applied evenly through your heel and forefoot. Hold for 5 seconds.

Core and upper legs

The **spinal extensors** and **transversus abdominis** engage isometrically, neither lengthening or shortening, to maintain an upright posture and support the motion. In your upper legs, the **hip flexors** and the **adductor magnus** also engage to support your body.

Spine
Spinal extensors
Transversus abdominis
Tensor fascia latae
Hip
Adductor magnus
Knee

STAGE TWO

Relax your foot, allowing it to return to the starting position. Repeat stages one and two.

Intrinsic muscles stretch

Medial arch descends

Foot core lengthens

Medial arch rises

Intrinsic foot muscles engage concentrically

Keep toes relaxed

LATERAL-INFERIOR VIEW

Abductor hallucis
Quadratus plantae
Abductor digiti minimi
Flexor d. m. brevis
Flexor hallucis brevis
Lumbricals

Foot

The **intrinsic muscles** of the foot shorten under tension as you draw the base of your big toe toward your heel. This concentric action strengthens and stabilizes your arch.

» CLOSER LOOK

The foot is an incredibly complex structure that can act as both a spring and a shock absorber during running (see pp.18–19). As a runner, it is well worth taking the time to understand its anatomy (see pp.22–23) and to strengthen its structures with targeted exercises like Foot Doming.

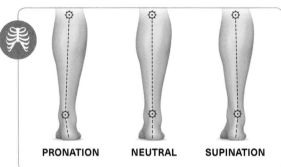

PRONATION **NEUTRAL** **SUPINATION**

Subtalar neutral

When the foot is midway between pronation and supination, it is in a neutral position, referred to as "subtalar neutral," because the ankle (subtalar) joint is aligned in its neutral zone. The talus stacks squarely on the calcaneus, allowing the tibia and fibula to sit squarely on top without any rotation at the ankle joint in the frontal plane. The knee should then be directly over the ankle if sitting. Aim for this position at the start of the exercise so you begin with the muscles in a midrange position.

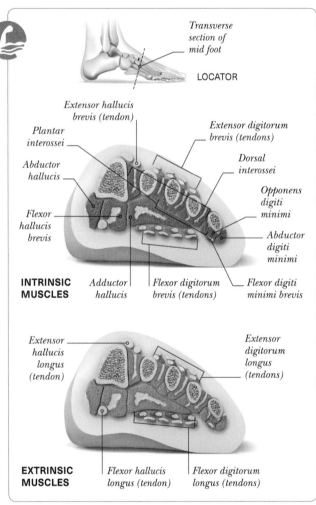

Transverse section of mid foot

LOCATOR

Extensor hallucis brevis (tendon)

Plantar interossei

Extensor digitorum brevis (tendons)

Abductor hallucis

Dorsal interossei

Opponens digiti minimi

Flexor hallucis brevis

Abductor digiti minimi

INTRINSIC MUSCLES *Adductor hallucis* *Flexor digitorum brevis (tendons)* *Flexor digiti minimi brevis*

Extensor hallucis longus (tendon)

Extensor digitorum longus (tendons)

EXTRINSIC MUSCLES *Flexor hallucis longus (tendon)* *Flexor digitorum longus (tendons)*

Intrinsic and extrinsic foot muscles

Foot doming strengthens both the intrinsic and extrinsic muscles of the foot. The extrinsic muscles originate from outside the foot, specifically the anterior, posterior, and lateral lower leg. They enable inversion, eversion, plantarflexion, and dorsiflexion of the ankle. The intrinsic muscles are located within the foot and are primarily responsible for stabilizing the foot and arch.

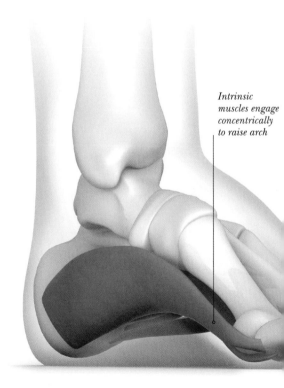

Intrinsic muscles engage concentrically to raise arch

STAGE ONE | ANTERIOR-MEDIAL VIEW

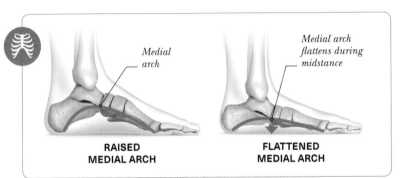

**RAISED
MEDIAL ARCH**

Medial arch

Medial arch flattens during midstance

**FLATTENED
MEDIAL ARCH**

Medial arch: the **shock absorber**

As the arch collapses in the midstance phase of running (see p.67), the medial longitudinal arch flattens and elongates. This acts as a shock-absorption mechanism, as the plantar fascia and intrinsic foot muscles generate tension to slow down this collapse and absorb energy from the weight of the body. The energy is then used to assist in propulsion as the foot resupinates and pushes off the ground. The foot provides up to 17 percent of the energy required to power a stride.

FOOT DOMING PROGRESSIONS
Dynamic Foot Doming

Progressions for this exercise (see p.100) involve increasing the amount of weight passing through the arch, adding movement, and mimicking the actions of running by using single-leg versions of the exercise. Add weight to your upper body by holding dumbbells and increasing the weight over time.

Lower yourself as if sitting in a chair

SQUAT

Perform Foot Doming on one leg at a time

SINGLE LEG

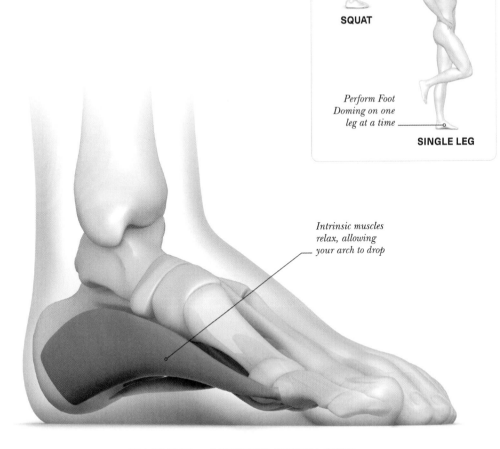

Relax your toes as you engage your muscles

Intrinsic muscles relax, allowing your arch to drop

STAGE TWO | ANTERIOR–MEDIAL VIEW

RESISTED TOE

Strong intrinsic muscles (see p.102) allow the foot to alternate between rigidity and flexibility, providing a stable foundation throughout the running cycle (see pp.66–69). This exercise strengthens the intrinsic muscles of the foot, as well as the extrinsic muscles and tendons supporting the medial and lateral longitudinal arches (see p.106).

THE **BIG PICTURE**

You will need a resistance band to perform this exercise. If you find it more comfortable, draw your nonfocus foot back to rest on your toes, with your focus foot planted on the floor throughout.

If new to this exercise, perform 3–4 sets of 10–12 repetitions. To advance, first increase the resistance (see p.99). Next, work through the following progressions to perform the exercise: while standing and while standing on one leg.

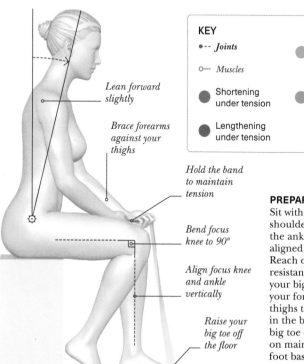

Lean forward slightly

Brace forearms against your thighs

Hold the band to maintain tension

Bend focus knee to 90°

Align focus knee and ankle vertically

Raise your big toe off the floor

KEY

●-- *Joints*

○— *Muscles*

● Shortening under tension

● Lengthening under tension

● Lengthening without tension (stretching)

● Held muscles without motion

PREPARATORY STAGE
Sit with your feet shoulder-width apart and the ankle of your focus leg aligned beneath your knee. Reach down and wrap the resistance band around your big toe, then brace your forearms against your thighs to maintain tension in the band and raise your big toe off the floor. Focus on maintaining a stable foot base. Keep both sides of your heel and forefoot in contact with the floor.

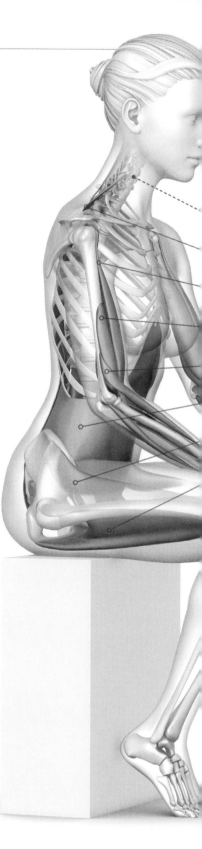

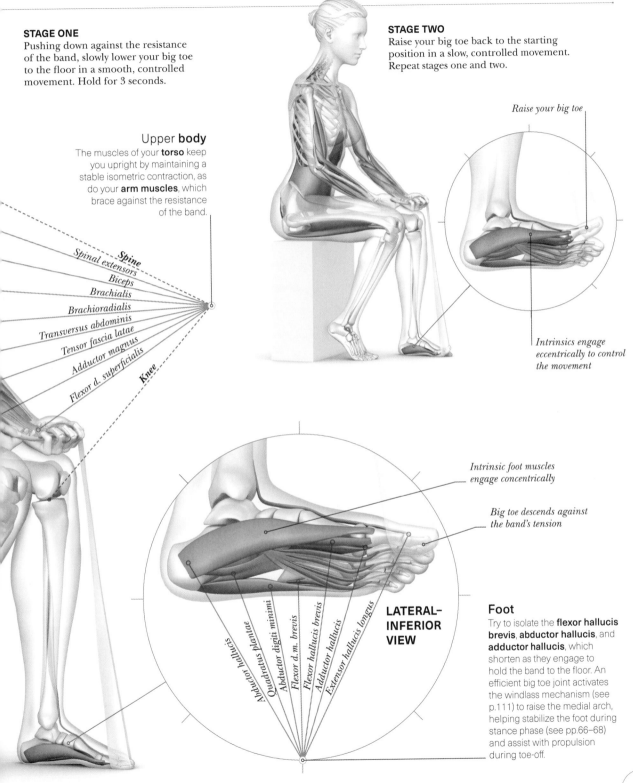

STAGE ONE
Pushing down against the resistance of the band, slowly lower your big toe to the floor in a smooth, controlled movement. Hold for 3 seconds.

STAGE TWO
Raise your big toe back to the starting position in a slow, controlled movement. Repeat stages one and two.

Raise your big toe

Intrinsics engage eccentrically to control the movement

Upper **body**
The muscles of your **torso** keep you upright by maintaining a stable isometric contraction, as do your **arm muscles**, which brace against the resistance of the band.

Spine
Spinal extensors
Biceps
Brachialis
Brachioradialis
Transversus abdominis
Tensor fascia latae
Adductor magnus
Flexor d. superficialis
Knee

Intrinsic foot muscles engage concentrically

Big toe descends against the band's tension

Abductor hallucis
Quadratus plantae
Abductor digiti minimi
Flexor d.m. brevis
Flexor hallucis brevis
Adductor hallucis
Extensor hallucis longus

LATERAL-INFERIOR VIEW

Foot
Try to isolate the **flexor hallucis brevis**, **abductor hallucis**, and **adductor hallucis**, which shorten as they engage to hold the band to the floor. An efficient big toe joint activates the windlass mechanism (see p.111) to raise the medial arch, helping stabilize the foot during stance phase (see pp.66–68) and assist with propulsion during toe-off.

❯❯ CLOSER LOOK

The toes are vital structures in themselves. The muscles that control them contribute to the overall capacity for power generation and shock absorption. Strengthening the individual muscles of the toes through exercises like Resisted Toe and its variations will give you a more stable and powerful base for running.

Big-toe **energy loss**

During the push-off phase in running, the big-toe joint bends, resulting in lost energy. The windlass mechanism (see p.111) limits this bending by resisting the movement. Some recent shoe designs include a carbon-fiber plate to reduce bending and instead transfer work to the ankle. While this has positive implications for performance, it increases stress elsewhere, possibly increasing injury risk.

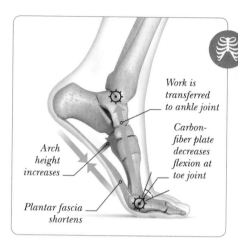

Work is transferred to ankle joint

Carbon-fiber plate decreases flexion at toe joint

Arch height increases

Plantar fascia shortens

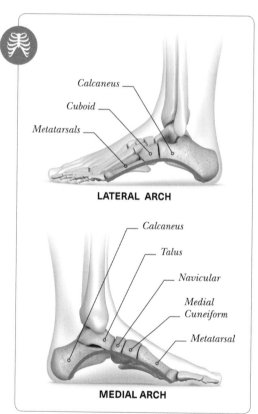

Calcaneus

Cuboid

Metatarsals

LATERAL ARCH

Calcaneus

Talus

Navicular

Medial Cuneiform

Metatarsal

MEDIAL ARCH

Strengthening the **arches**

The two longitudinal arches of the foot are composed of different sets of bones and are supported by different muscles (see p.22). Depending on which variation of the exercise you perform (see opposite), you strengthen your medial arch (by exercising your big toe), your lateral arch (by working your fifth toe), or both (by working any of your other toes).

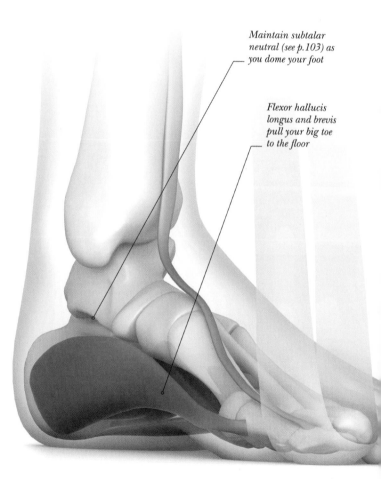

Maintain subtalar neutral (see p.103) as you dome your foot

Flexor hallucis longus and brevis pull your big toe to the floor

STAGE ONE | ANTERIOR–MEDIAL VIEW

Hallux valgus (bunion)

A bunion is a painful bony bump that develops on the medial foot at the big-toe joint, as pressure on the joint causes the big toe to bend inward. This deformity gradually increases, making it painful to wear certain shoes or to run. Bunions may be caused by narrow shoes or biomechanics (abducted feet). Strengthening the feet with targeted foot exercises may help prevent and treat bunions.

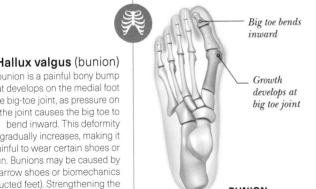

Big toe bends inward

Growth develops at big toe joint

BUNION

RESISTED TOE VARIATIONS
Individual toes

Repeat the exercise with toes 2–5 to strengthen different intrinsic foot muscles. For example, when carried out with your second toe (shown below), the flexor digitorum brevis, lumbricals, and quadratus plantae are activated. When performed with your fifth toe, the abductor digiti minimi is activated, which strengthens your lateral longitudinal arch.

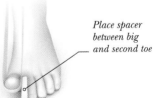

Wrap band around target toe

Misaligned big toe

If your big toe does not align neutrally but points inward (as may be the case with a bunion, see above left), use a toe spacer between your big toe and second toe. This brings the big toe muscles to the optimal length for exercising, and strengthening the muscles may improve alignment.

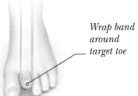

Place spacer between big and second toe

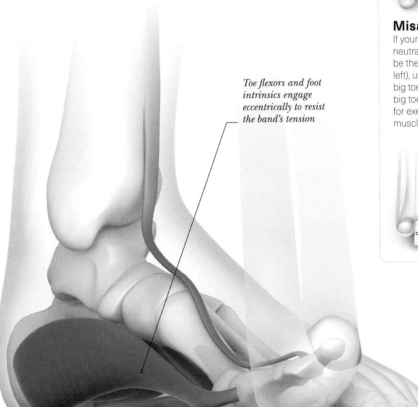

Toe flexors and foot intrinsics engage eccentrically to resist the band's tension

STAGE TWO | ANTERIOR-MEDIAL VIEW

HEEL DROP

The plantar flexor muscles and Achilles tendon absorb considerable impact forces during the loading phase of the running cycle and also generate powerful propulsion forces for toe-off (see pp.18–19). Heel Drop strengthens this muscle group.

THE BIG PICTURE

You will need a low exercise step (see p.99) for Heel Drop, or use the bottom step of a staircase. During the exercise, your forefeet should remain in contact with the step from the ball of the foot to the tips of the toes only. Hold onto the back of a chair or a stair railing for support. Focus on the calves and Achilles tendon as you raise and drop the heels.

If new to the exercise, perform 3 sets of 10–12 repetitions. To progress, work through the following progressions: add weights (see p.99) and reduce to 3–4 sets of 6–8 repetitions; practice on one leg; increase the speed of the movement.

Caution

If you have a history of insertional Achilles pain or bursitis, perform this exercise on the floor and stop the heel drop at the neutral (flat feet) position to avoid taking the ankles into dorsiflexion.

KEY

- •— *Joints*
- ○— *Muscles*
- ● Shortening under tension
- ● Lengthening under tension
- ● Lengthening without tension (stretching)
- ● Held muscles without motion

Semispinalis capitis

Deltoids

Spinal extensors

Pectoralis major

Brachialis

Triceps medial head

Elbow

Latissimus dorsi

Transversus abdominis

Brachioradialis

Wrist

Flexor digitorum profundus

Upper **body** holding the railing to stabilize your body to avoid having to work on your balance during the exercise. Your body should be stable while your calves perform this eccentric work.

Use the **arm** holding the railing to stabilize your body to avoid having to work on your balance during the exercise.

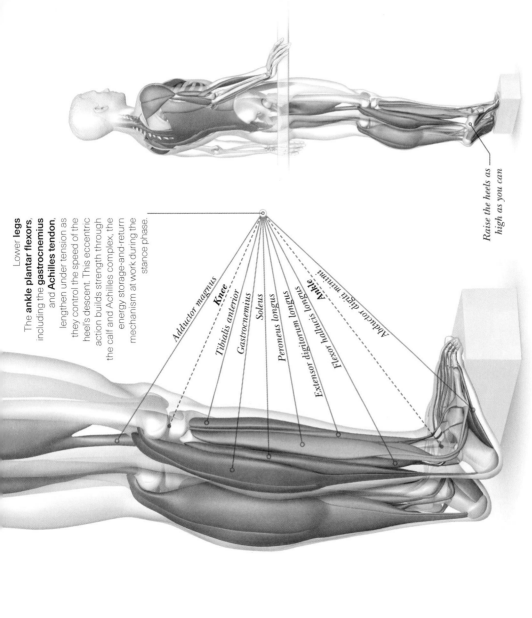

Lower **legs**
The **ankle plantar flexors**, including the **gastrocnemius** and **Achilles tendon**, lengthen under tension as they control the speed of the heel's descent. This eccentric action builds strength through the calf and Achilles complex, the energy storage-and-return mechanism at work during the stance phase.

Adductor magnus

Knee

Tibialis anterior

Gastrocnemius

Soleus

Peroneus longus

Extensor digitorum longus

Ankle

Flexor hallucis longus

Abductor digiti minimi

Raise the heels as high as you can

STAGE TWO
As soon as your heels reach their lowest point, immediately raise them again. Using a slow, controlled movement (taking 3 seconds), return them to their topmost position. Hold at the top for 2 seconds. Repeat stages one and two.

STAGE ONE
Slowly (taking 3 seconds) drop your heels down as far as they will go in a smooth, controlled movement.

Maintain an upright posture

Hold a railing for support

Keep the knees straight

Forefeet are planted firmly on the step

PREPARATORY STAGE
Stand with the balls of your feet on the step, feet just less than hip-width apart. Ensure your weight is distributed evenly across the forefeet. Keep your ankles neutral and your feet parallel to the floor. Now raise your heels as high as possible.

» CLOSER LOOK

Heel Drop and its variations activate the calf, Achilles tendon, and plantar fascia. If you invest time in strengthening any one area of your body, make it this group of muscles, which contributes roughly half the work required for each step. Included here are variations of the Heel Drop exercise that work the soleus muscle and the plantar fascia.

HEEL DROP VARIATION

Seated Heel Drop

This version of Heel Drop works the soleus, which bears loads of up to eight times your body weight during running. Place your forefeet on the step, bend your knees to 90°, and lay a cushion on your lap with a weighted barbell on top. Now lower and raise your heels as in the main exercise, ending the drop stage when your heels touch the floor or reach their lowest point. Perform 3 sets of 10–12 reps. To progress, add weight (see p.99) and reduce to 3–4 sets of 6–8 reps.

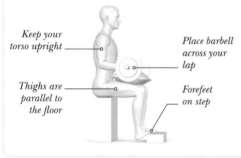

Keep your torso upright

Place barbell across your lap

Thighs are parallel to the floor

Forefeet on step

Shape of the **arch**
During the exercise, try to maintain a subtalar neutral ankle position (see p.103) and an engaged medial longitudinal arch (see p.107) as you raise and lower the heels. This activates both the intrinsic and extrinsic foot muscles (see p.102). Avoid allowing your ankle to roll in and collapse your arch.

Engage medial arch as you raise and lower heels

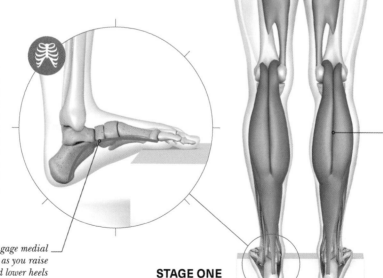

Stand tall, gaze forward, and keep your hips and knees straight

Plantarflexor muscles engage eccentrically to lower heels

**STAGE ONE
POSTERIOR VIEW**

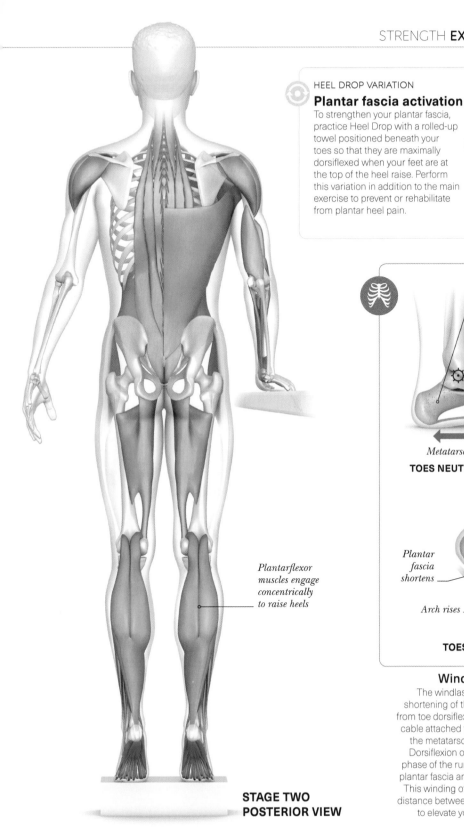

Plantarflexor muscles engage concentrically to raise heels

**STAGE TWO
POSTERIOR VIEW**

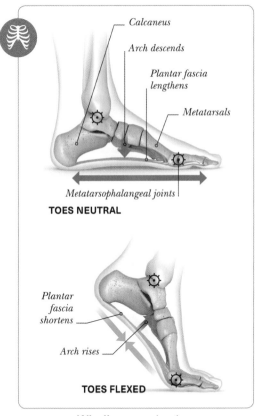

HEEL DROP VARIATION
Plantar fascia activation
To strengthen your plantar fascia, practice Heel Drop with a rolled-up towel positioned beneath your toes so that they are maximally dorsiflexed when your feet are at the top of the heel raise. Perform this variation in addition to the main exercise to prevent or rehabilitate from plantar heel pain.

Place a rolled-up towel under your toes

Calcaneus

Arch descends

Plantar fascia lengthens

Metatarsals

Metatarsophalangeal joints

TOES NEUTRAL

Plantar fascia shortens

Arch rises

TOES FLEXED

Windlass mechanism
The windlass mechanism describes the shortening of the longitudinal arch that results from toe dorsiflexion. The plantar fascia acts like a cable attached to the calcaneus at one end and the metatarsophalangeal joints at the other. Dorsiflexion of the toe during the propulsive phase of the running cycle (see p.68) winds the plantar fascia around the head of the metatarsal. This winding of the plantar fascia shortens the distance between the calcaneus and metatarsals to elevate your medial longitudinal arch.

ANKLE TURN OUT

This exercise strengthens the lateral stabilizers of the lower leg—the ankle evertors. During the main stage, as the ankle is inverting, the evertors engage, working against the band's tension to resist the ankle turning in so that the movement is smooth and controlled.

THE BIG PICTURE

You will need a resistance band for this exercise. Secure it at ankle height and position your chair so the band approaches your focus foot medially. It should be taut enough to work the ankle evertors during stage one. During the exercise, isolate the movement to your ankle. Do not allow your leg to move.

If new to this exercise, perform 3 sets of 15–20 reps on each side with light resistance. To progress, increase the resistance (see p.99) and reduce to 3–4 sets of 6–8 reps.

Core
Engage your **transversus abdominis** to maintain a neutral and stable spine. The **iliopsoas** and **adductor muscles** stabilize the hip to maintain a firm anchor for the lower leg muscles.

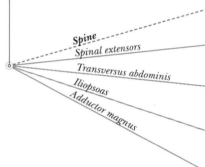

Spine
Spinal extensors
Transversus abdominis
Iliopsoas
Adductor magnus

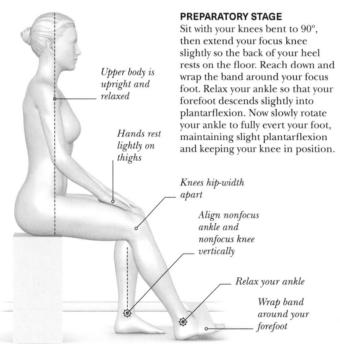

Upper body is upright and relaxed

Hands rest lightly on thighs

Knees hip-width apart

Align nonfocus ankle and nonfocus knee vertically

Relax your ankle

Wrap band around your forefoot

PREPARATORY STAGE
Sit with your knees bent to 90°, then extend your focus knee slightly so the back of your heel rests on the floor. Reach down and wrap the band around your focus foot. Relax your ankle so that your forefoot descends slightly into plantarflexion. Now slowly rotate your ankle to fully evert your foot, maintaining slight plantarflexion and keeping your knee in position.

Lower leg
The **peroneus longus** and **peroneus brevis** work eccentrically, lengthening as they slow down the inversion of the foot. Strong **ankle evertors** stabilize the lateral ankle, which helps prevent ankle inversion sprains—the most common type—and promotes rehabilitation from them.

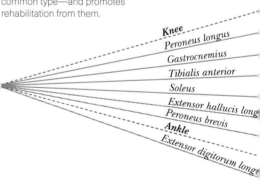

Knee
Peroneus longus
Gastrocnemius
Tibialis anterior
Soleus
Extensor hallucis long
Peroneus brevis
Ankle
Extensor digitorum long

STAGE ONE
Slowly (over 3 seconds) rotate your ankle to bring your foot into full inversion. Use a slow, controlled scooping motion, keeping your foot close to the floor.

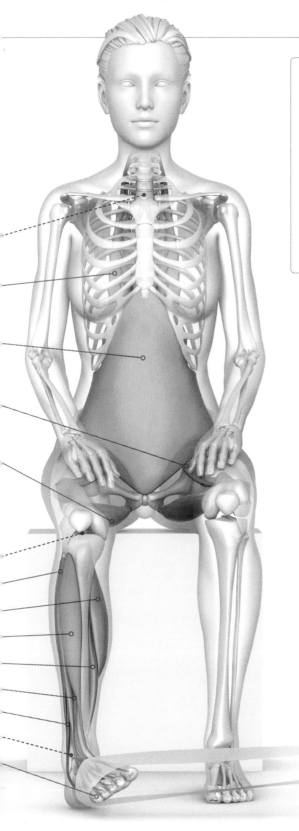

KEY

●-- *Joints*

○— *Muscles*

● Shortening under tension

● Lengthening under tension

● Lengthening without tension (stretching)

● Held muscles without motion

Keep your knee still while you rotate your ankle

Rotate at your ankle

Move your foot in a scooping motion

STAGE TWO

Take 2 seconds to return your foot into eversion in a smooth scooping motion. Repeat stages one and two.

ANKLE TURN IN

This exercise strengthens the ankle invertors, the medial stabilizers of the lower leg. During the main stage, as the ankle is everting, the invertors engage, working against the band's tension to resist the ankle turning out so that the movement is smooth and controlled.

THE **BIG PICTURE**

You will need a resistance band for this exercise. Secure it at ankle height and position your chair so the band approaches your focus foot laterally. As with Ankle Turn Out (see pp.112–113), keep the movement within your ankle joint. The knee of your focus leg remains still throughout.

If new to this exercise, perform 3 sets of 15–20 reps with light resistance. To progress, increase the resistance (see p.99) and reduce to 3–4 sets of 6–8 reps, then move on to the progression shown on p.116.

Core
Engage your **transversus abdominis** to maintain a neutral and stable spine. The **iliopsoas** and **adductor muscles** stabilize the hip to maintain a firm anchor for the lower leg muscles.

Spine
Spinal extensors
Transversus abdominis
Iliopsoas
Adductor magnus

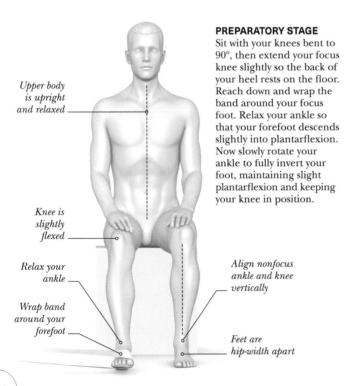

Upper body is upright and relaxed

Knee is slightly flexed

Relax your ankle

Wrap band around your forefoot

Align nonfocus ankle and knee vertically

Feet are hip-width apart

PREPARATORY STAGE
Sit with your knees bent to 90°, then extend your focus knee slightly so the back of your heel rests on the floor. Reach down and wrap the band around your focus foot. Relax your ankle so that your forefoot descends slightly into plantarflexion. Now slowly rotate your ankle to fully invert your foot, maintaining slight plantarflexion and keeping your knee in position.

Lower **leg**
The **tibialis posterior** works eccentrically, lengthening as it controls the eversion of the foot. This muscle is important for controlling pronation. It helps stabilize the arch through pronation during the stance phase of running (see pp.66–68).

Knee
Peroneus longus
Gastrocnemius
Tibialis anterior
Soleus
Extensor digitorum lon
Peroneus brevis
Ankle
Extensor hallucis longus

STAGE ONE
Slowly (over 3 seconds) rotate your ankle to bring your foot into full eversion. Use a slow, controlled scooping motion, keeping your foot close to the floor.

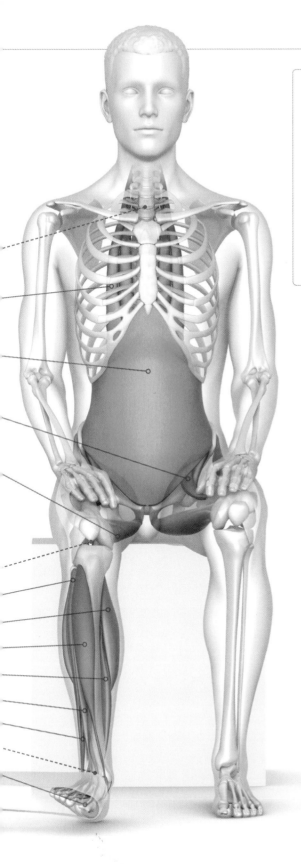

KEY

•-- *Joints*

○— *Muscles*

● Shortening under tension

● Lengthening under tension

● Lengthening without tension (stretching)

● Held muscles without motion

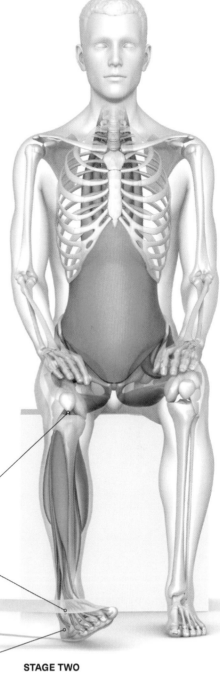

Keep your knee still while you rotate your ankle

Rotate at your ankle

Move your foot in a scooping motion

STAGE TWO
Take 2 seconds to return your foot in a smooth scooping motion to inversion. Repeat stages one and two.

» CLOSER LOOK

The muscles of the medial and lateral lower leg stabilize your ankle joint when you run across rough terrain. They also support your arch from above, especially during the early loading phase (see pp.66–68). Practice Ankle Turn Out in conjunction with Ankle Turn In to develop all-around strength and stability in your lower limbs.

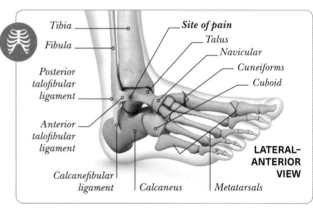

Tibia

Fibula

Posterior talofibular ligament

Anterior talofibular ligament

Calcanefibular ligament

Site of pain

Talus

Navicular

Cuneiforms

Cuboid

Calcaneus

Metatarsals

LATERAL-ANTERIOR VIEW

Relax tibialis anterior and allow your ankle to remain slightly plantarflexed

Peroneus longus and brevis engage concentrically to evert ankle

Chronic ankle instability

Approximately one in five people with acute ankle sprains go on to develop chronic ankle instability. Following an acute sprain, deficits in balance, strength, and reaction time typically occur. These can result in recurrent sprains if the condition is not rehabilitated appropriately. Some runners also report impingement pain in the anterior ankle joint. Strength training targeting the ankle invertors and evertors may help runners avoid this recurring condition or recover from it successfully.

Muscles that evert the ankle

The ankle evertors help stabilize the lateral ankle and protect against ankle sprains, which are typically inversion sprains. This is important when running on uneven terrain such as trails and cambered surfaces (see p.51).

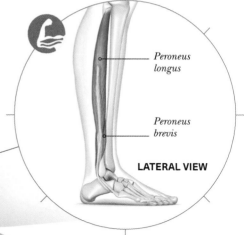

Peroneus longus

Peroneus brevis

LATERAL VIEW

ANKLE TURN OUT | STAGE ONE | ANTERIOR-LATERAL VIEW

ANKLE TURN OUT VARIATION

Eccentric Eversion on Step

Stand on the edge of a step with the medial half of your foot off the step. Raise the other foot, holding a railing for support if necessary. Slowly (over 3 seconds) roll onto the lateral side of your foot so the medial side is higher. Hold for 2 seconds, then slowly (over 3 seconds) evert the ankle so the medial side is lower. Raise the medial side again to complete 1 rep. Perform 3 sets of 10–12 reps on each leg. To progress, hold a dumbbell in the opposite hand and reduce to 3–4 sets of 6–8 reps.

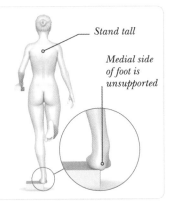

Stand tall

Medial side of foot is unsupported

Do not allow tibialis anterior to dorsiflex your foot; keep ankle slightly plantarflexed

Tibialis posterior should be the prime mover for this exercise

Muscles that invert the ankle

The ankle invertors are extrinsic foot muscles (see p.102) that control arch collapse. The tibialis posterior attaches into the medial longitudinal arch and slows down arch collapse during the stance phase of running (see pp.66–69). Bearing large loads during running, this muscle is vulnerable to posterior tibial tendon dysfunction. Strength training may help prevent the condition.

Tibialis anterior

Tibialis posterior

MEDIAL VIEW

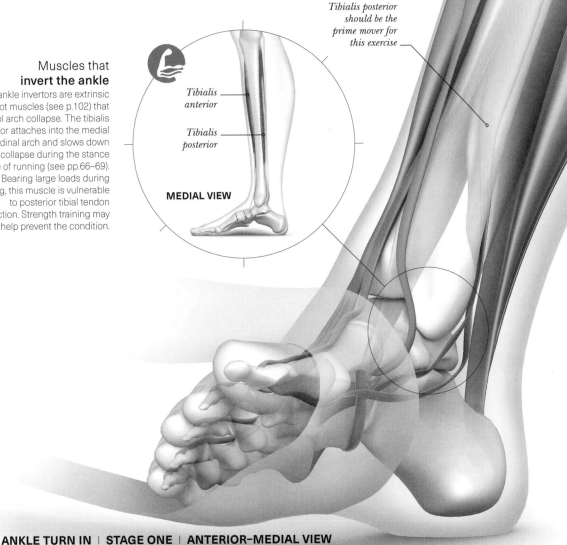

ANKLE TURN IN | STAGE ONE | ANTERIOR-MEDIAL VIEW

HIP HIKE

Hip Hike strengthens the hip abductors, which play an important role in maintaining stability of the pelvis during running. Weak or poorly recruited hip abductors have been linked to a number of running injuries such as iliotibial band pain (see p.61) and patellofemoral pain (see p.57).

THE **BIG PICTURE**

The glutes are your target here. Use the stance-leg glutes to raise and lower the opposite hip during the exercise. Try not to rely on the abdominal muscles on the nonstance side to lower the pelvis.

If new to this exercise, perform 3 sets of 10–12 reps on each side. Once comfortable, add weights (for example, hold a dumbbell on the opposite side of the body to the stance leg) and reduce to 3–4 sets of 6–8 reps.

Upper body and hip

Your **hip abductors,** especially the **gluteus medius,** control the contralateral pelvic drop (CPD, see p.73). Strength in these muscles helps during the early loading stage of the running cycle (see p.66), when the ground reaction force produces a torque (see p.48) around the hip that causes CPD. Eccentric control of the hip abductors determines the magnitude and rate of the CPD. The **spinal extensors** of the lower back also help control the descent of the hips.

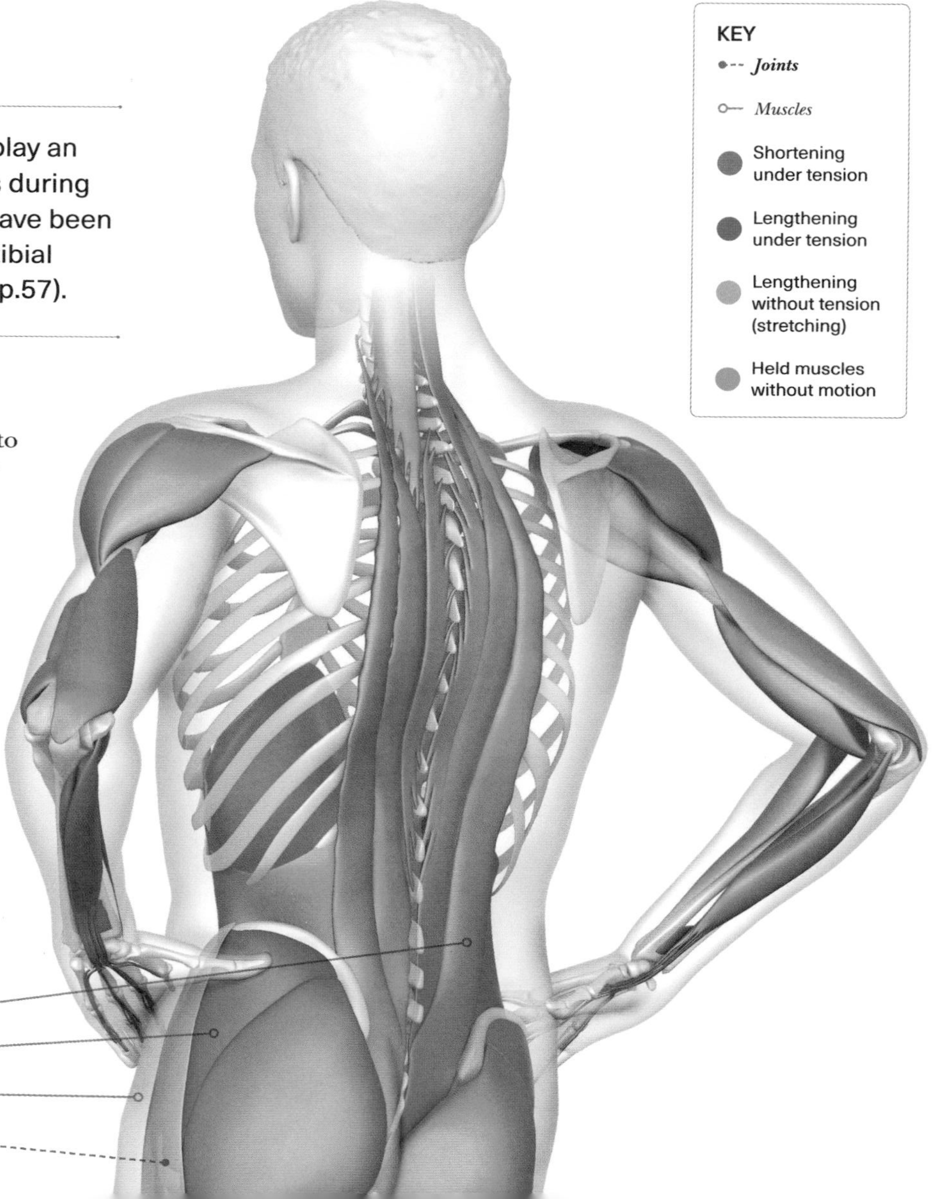

Spinal extensors

Gluteus medius

Tensor fascia latae

Hip

Gluteus maximus

Adductor magnus

KEY

• - - *Joints*

○— *Muscles*

● Shortening under tension

● Lengthening under tension

● Lengthening without tension (stretching)

● Held muscles without motion

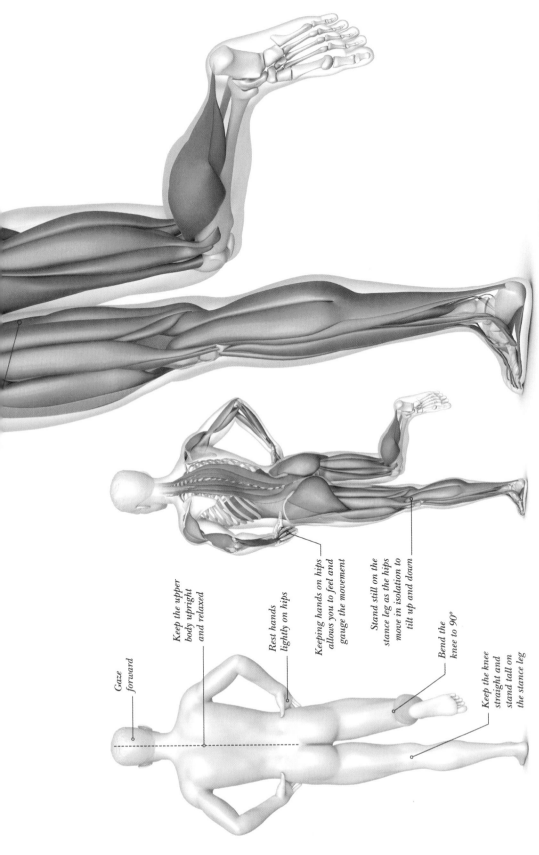

PREPARATORY STAGE

Stand tall with hands on hips. Keeping your knees aligned, bend one knee to 90° and raise your heel behind you so that your shin is parallel to the floor. Relax your foot. Ensure your hips are level and your weight is evenly distributed across the stance foot.

Gaze forward

Keep the upper body upright and relaxed

Rest hands lightly on hips

Keeping hands on hips allows you to feel and gauge the movement

Stand still on the stance leg as the hips move in isolation to tilt up and down

Bend the knee to 90°

Keep the knee straight and stand tall on the stance leg

STAGE ONE

Slowly (over 3 seconds) raise the nonstance hip so that your pelvis is lower on the stance side. Hold for 2 seconds.

STAGE TWO

Slowly (over 3 seconds) lower the raised hip as far as it will go so that it is now higher on the stance side. Repeat stages one and two.

119

STEP DOWN

The quadriceps and hip abductors are among the main muscle groups used in running. One important role they play is to help control knee alignment. Training these muscles with exercises like Step Down increases strength and control and reduces your risk of injury.

THE BIG PICTURE

You will need an exercise step that is 4–6 in (10–15 cm) high for this exercise. Note that the focus leg is the stance leg, not the stepping leg. Ensure it is fully supported on the step. (Your toes should not extend over the edge.) Concentrate on the stance-leg quads and glutes as you bend and straighten your knee. Also, pay attention to the position of the stance knee throughout the exercise; it should not move medially. Maintaining its position in the frontal plane (see p.10) is important in this exercise. Do not transfer any weight onto the stepping leg when it reaches the floor. Simply touch down with your heel before you raise your leg again.

If you are new to this exercise, perform 3 sets of 10–12 reps on each side. To progress, add weight (see p.99) and reduce to 3–4 sets of 6–8 reps. Then move on to Single Leg Hop (see pp.154–155) and Box Jump (see pp.150–151).

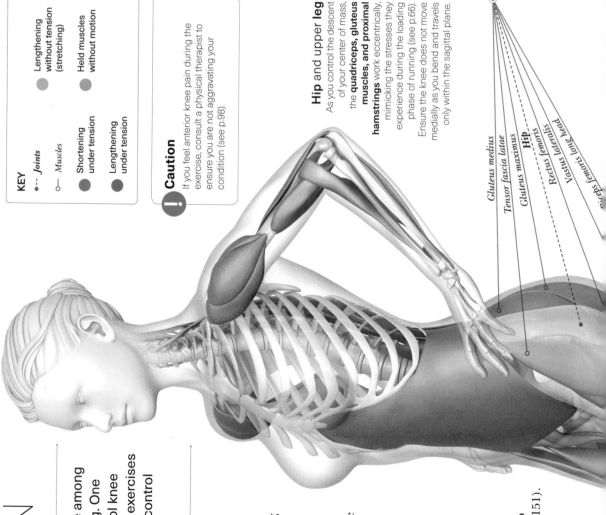

KEY

- ●-- *Joints*
- ○— *Muscles*
- ● Shortening under tension
- ● Lengthening under tension
- ● Lengthening without tension (stretching)
- ● Held muscles without motion

⚠ Caution

If you feel anterior knee pain during the exercise, consult a physical therapist to ensure you are not aggravating your condition (see p.98).

Hip and upper leg

As you control the descent of your center of mass, the **quadriceps, gluteus muscles, and proximal hamstrings** work eccentrically, mimicking the stresses they experience during the loading phase of running (see p.66). Ensure the knee does not move medially as you bend and travels only within the sagittal plane.

Gluteus medius
Tensor fascia latae
Gluteus maximus
Hip
Rectus femoris
Vastus lateralis
Biceps femoris long head

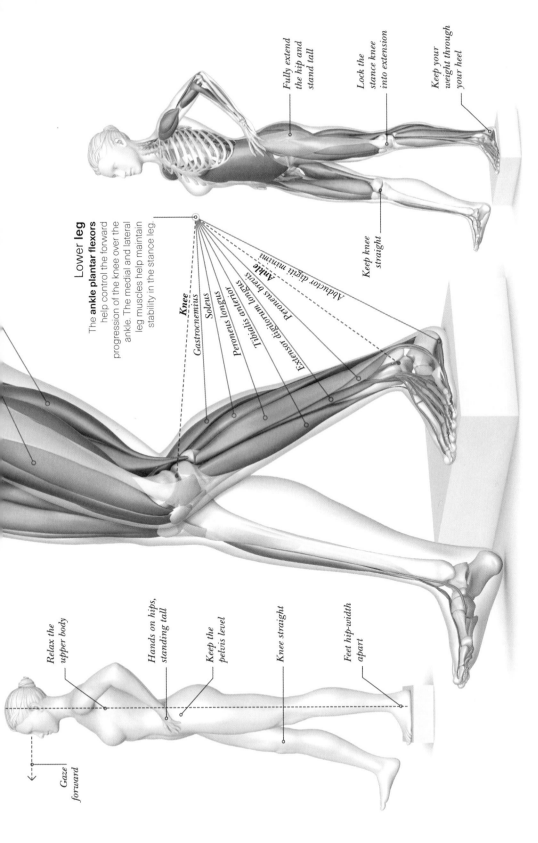

Lower leg

The **ankle plantar flexors** help control the forward progression of the knee over the ankle. The medial and lateral leg muscles help maintain stability in the stance leg.

Fully extend the hip and stand tall

Lock the stance knee into extension

Keep your weight through your heel

Keep knee straight

Knee
Gastrocnemius
Soleus
Peroneus longus
Tibialis anterior
Extensor digitorum longus
Peroneus brevis
Ankle
Abductor digiti minimi

Relax the upper body

Hands on hips, standing tall

Keep the pelvis level

Knee straight

Feet hip-width apart

Gaze forward

STAGE TWO
Slowly (taking 3 seconds) straighten the stance leg to return to the starting position. Hold this position for 2 seconds. Repeat stages one and two.

STAGE ONE
Slowly (taking 3 seconds) bend the stance knee to lower the "stepping" foot to the floor, touching it lightly with the heel. Keep the weight through the heel of your stance foot throughout the movement, and keep your hips level.

PREPARATORY STAGE
Stand tall on the step, hands on hips. Shift your weight into the stance leg. Now reach out in front of you with the nonstance leg as though about to step down. Ensure you keep your hips level.

STEP UP

This exercise offers a great method of strengthening the quadriceps and glutes, which are muscles that play an important role during the propulsion stage of running.

Caution

If you feel anterior knee pain during the exercise, consult a physical therapist to ensure you are not aggravating your condition (see p.98).

THE **BIG PICTURE**

You will need an exercise step at least 12 in (30 cm) high for Step Up. The focus leg is the one that remains on the step. Ensure it is fully supported on the step and that your toes do not extend over the edge. This exercise involves the coordinated movement of your arms and legs. The arms adopt a running position. Then, as you shift your weight onto the focus leg, raise the opposite arm to the raised leg, as you would if running.

If new to this exercise, perform 3 sets of 10–12 reps on each side. To progress, add weight (see p.99) and reduce to 3–4 sets of 6–8 reps.

Upper **body**

Swing your arms, raising the opposite arm to help drive your body up, just as you would for running. The **core** and **back** **muscles** engage to support the upward driving movement.

Semispinalis capitis
Spinal extensors
Deltoids
Pectoralis major
Biceps
Brachialis
Triceps
Serratus anterior
Spine
Latissimus dorsi
Transversus abdominis

Hip and leg

As you step up, focus on the **glutes** and **quads**. Their concentric work here mimics their action during the propulsive part of the running cycle (see p.68). Strengthening the concentric function of the **glutes**, **proximal hamstrings** and **quadriceps** as you fully extend the hip and knee improves their ability to produce an explosive propulsion force for toe-off.

Gluteus medius
Iliopsoas
Hip
Tensor fascia latae

KEY

- ● - - *Joints*
- ○— *Muscles*
- ● Shortening under tension
- ● Lengthening under tension
- ● Lengthening without tension (stretching)
- ● Held muscles without motion

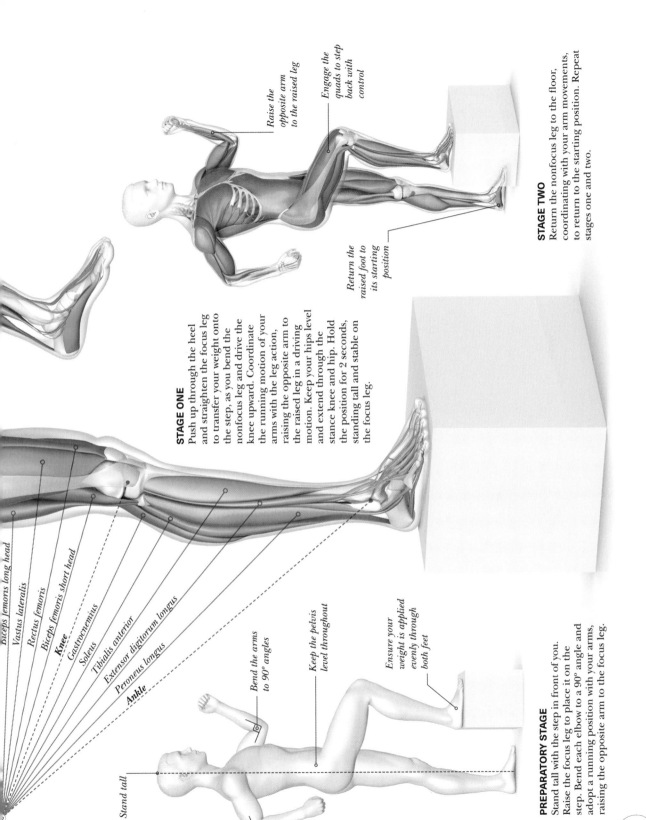

Raise the opposite arm to the raised leg

Engage the quads to step back with control

STAGE TWO
Return the nonfocus leg to the floor, coordinating with your arm movements, to return to the starting position. Repeat stages one and two.

Return the raised foot to its starting position

STAGE ONE
Push up through the heel and straighten the focus leg to transfer your weight onto the step, as you bend the nonfocus leg and drive the knee upward. Coordinate the running motion of your arms with the leg action, raising the opposite arm to the raised leg in a driving motion. Keep your hips level and extend through the stance knee and hip. Hold the position for 2 seconds, standing tall and stable on the focus leg.

Biceps femoris long head
Vastus lateralis
Rectus femoris
Biceps femoris short head
Knee
Gastrocnemius
Soleus
Tibialis anterior
Extensor digitorum longus
Peroneus longus
Ankle

Bend the arms to 90° angles

Keep the pelvis level throughout

Ensure your weight is applied evenly through both feet

Stand tall

PREPARATORY STAGE
Stand tall with the step in front of you. Raise the focus leg to place it on the step. Bend each elbow to a 90° angle and adopt a running position with your arms, raising the opposite arm to the focus leg.

» CLOSER LOOK

The movements involved in these exercises mimic the early loading (Step Down) and terminal stance (Step Up) phases of running. Learning how to control these movements and building strength for them will improve your efficiency as a runner.

STEP DOWN VARIATION
Single Leg Squat

This exercise strengthens the glutes, quads, and hip abductors. Stand tall with hands on hips. Raise one foot and bend your knee to 90°, keeping it aligned with the stance knee. Slowly (over 3 seconds) bend the stance knee to lower yourself, then slowly (over 2 seconds) straighten it to return to the starting position. Perform 3 sets of 10–12 reps. To progress, add weight (see p.99) and reduce to 3–4 sets of 6–8 reps. If you feel anterior knee pain during the exercise, consult a physical therapist (see p.98).

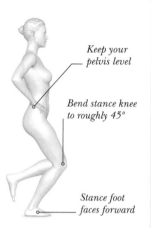

Keep your pelvis level

Bend stance knee to roughly 45°

Stance foot faces forward

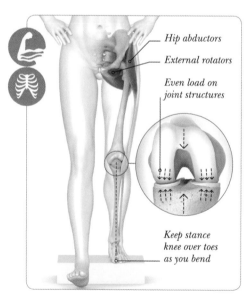

Hip abductors

External rotators

Even load on joint structures

Keep stance knee over toes as you bend

Knee alignment
When performing Step Down, it is important to maintain the alignment of the stance knee. It should move primarily within the sagittal plane (see p.10) as you descend and rise. Engage the hip abductors and external rotators to avoid the valgus collapse of your knee (see p.73) toward the midline.

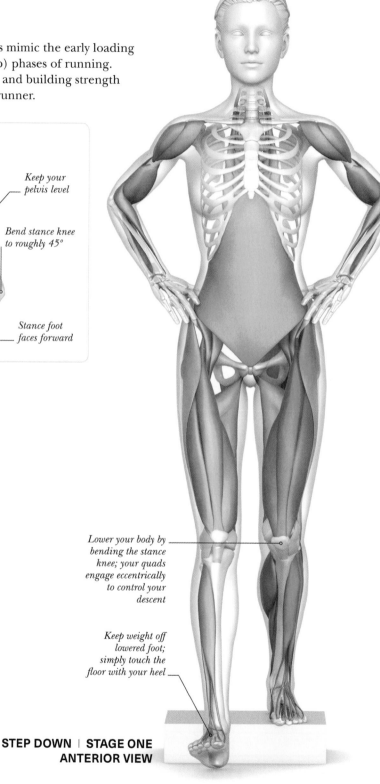

Lower your body by bending the stance knee; your quads engage eccentrically to control your descent

Keep weight off lowered foot; simply touch the floor with your heel

**STEP DOWN | STAGE ONE
ANTERIOR VIEW**

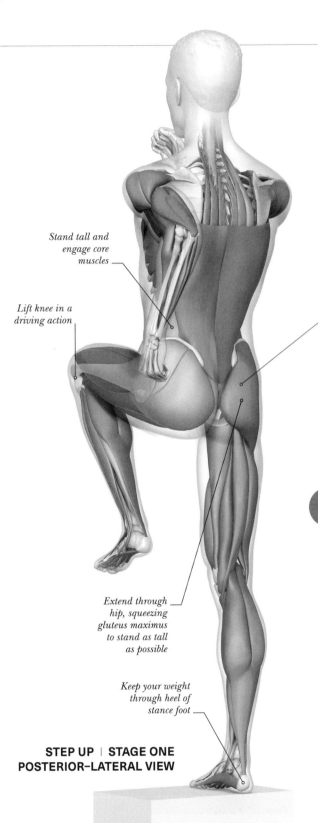

Stand tall and
engage core
muscles

Lift knee in a
driving action

Extend through
hip, squeezing
gluteus maximus
to stand as tall
as possible

Keep your weight
through heel of
stance foot

**STEP UP | STAGE ONE
POSTERIOR-LATERAL VIEW**

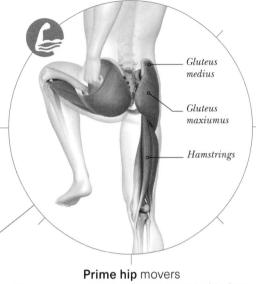

*Gluteus
medius*

*Gluteus
maxiumus*

Hamstrings

Prime hip movers

When we run, the hip extensors produce much of the force
required to propel our body forward. Given their proximity to
the axis of rotation of the hip, the glutes should be the prime
mover for this action, with the hamstrings working secondarily.
Regularly spending long hours seated lengthens the glutes
and keeps them from being recruited, placing undue strain on
the hamstrings. The Step Up exercise targets the glutes, which
results in better recruitment of these muscles.

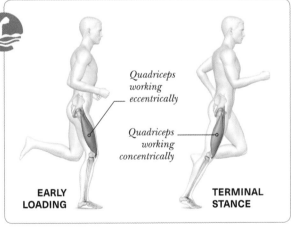

*Quadriceps
working
eccentrically*

*Quadriceps
working
concentrically*

**EARLY
LOADING**

**TERMINAL
STANCE**

Role of the **quadricep muscles**

During the loading phase of running (see p.66), the knee flexes
to absorb the ground reaction force, while the quads work
eccentrically to control the rate of this flexion. During the
propulsive phase (see p.68), they work concentrically to extend
the knee and drive the body forward. These actions are
mimicked during the Step Down (eccentric) and Step Up
(concentric) exercises, which target the quads to improve their
performance in running and help avoid injury.

125

STANDING
HIP ROTATION

Performing this exercise regularly strengthens the hip abductors and external rotators. These muscles provide stability at the hip during running, which helps prevent injury and improve running form.

THE **BIG PICTURE**

The rotation of the torso in this exercise is achieved by using the hip muscles of the stance leg, not by turning out the opposite hip. Focus on using the glutes (located at the side of the hip) of the stance leg as you rotate. Ensure the knee of the stance leg stands tall and faces forward throughout the exercise. Keep the opposite hip flexed to 90° and your pelvis square with your chest so that they turn as a unit. Keep your hips level throughout.

Perform 3 sets of 15–20 repetitions on each side. Then move on to Single Leg Ball Squat with pelvic rotation (see pp.136–139).

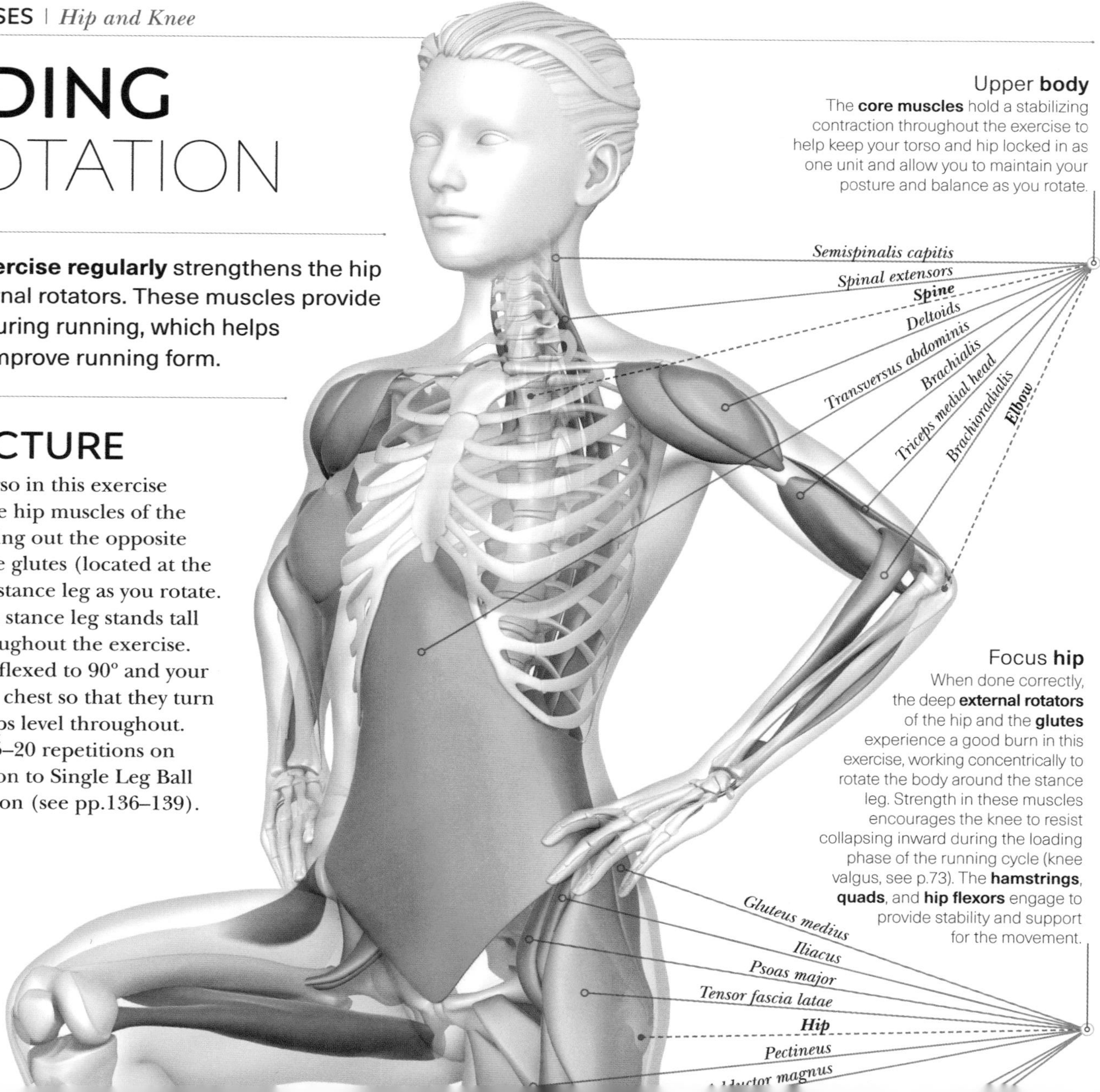

Upper **body**

The **core muscles** hold a stabilizing contraction throughout the exercise to help keep your torso and hip locked in as one unit and allow you to maintain your posture and balance as you rotate.

Semispinalis capitis
Spinal extensors
Spine
Deltoids
Brachiodialis
Triceps medial head
Brachioradialis
Elbow
Transversus abdominis

Focus **hip**

When done correctly, the deep **external rotators** of the hip and the **glutes** experience a good burn in this exercise, working concentrically to rotate the body around the stance leg. Strength in these muscles encourages the knee to resist collapsing inward during the loading phase of the running cycle (knee valgus, see p.73). The **hamstrings**, **quads**, and **hip flexors** engage to provide stability and support for the movement.

Gluteus medius
Iliacus
Psoas major
Tensor fascia latae
Hip
Pectineus
Adductor magnus

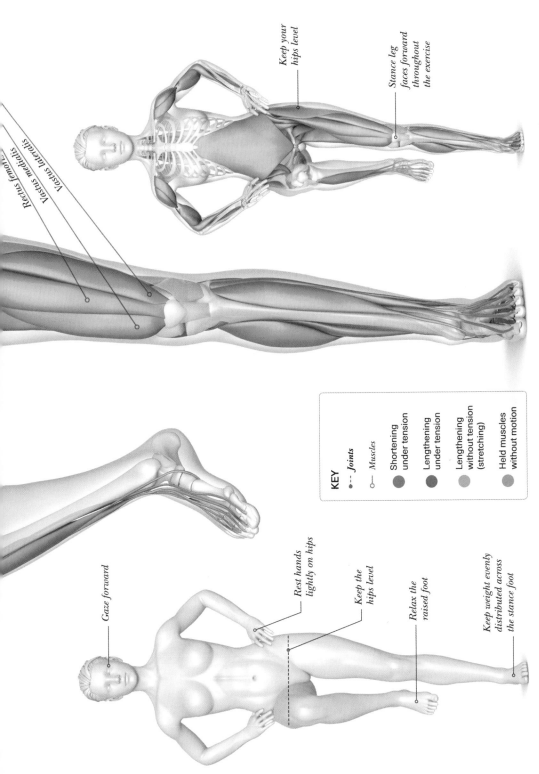

Rectus femoris

Vastus medialis

Vastus lateralis

Keep your hips level

Stance leg faces forward throughout the exercise

KEY

●-- *Joints*

○— *Muscles*

● Shortening under tension

● Lengthening under tension

● Lengthening without tension (stretching)

● Held muscles without motion

STAGE ONE

Using the glute muscles of the stance hip, slowly rotate your pelvis and torso in the direction of the raised leg. Keep the torso locked in with the pelvis so they turn as a unit. Ensure the stance leg does not turn in. Go as far as your hip range of motion allows. You may feel a stretch through the anterior hip during this stage.

STAGE TWO

Return your torso and pelvis back to the starting position as shown in the preparatory stage. Repeat stages one and two.

PREPARATORY STAGE

Stand tall with hands on hips. Raise one knee in front of you so that your thigh is parallel to the floor, keeping your hips level.

Gaze forward

Rest hands lightly on hips

Keep the hips level

Relax the raised foot

Keep weight evenly distributed across the stance foot

» CLOSER LOOK

Due to the ball-and-socket configuration of the hip joint (see p.26), rotations occur in all three planes, enabling a broad range of movement. The hip muscles play a key role in controlling these movements, as well as in absorbing the GRF (see pp.46–47) and generating power for push-off.

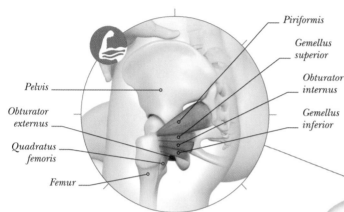

Piriformis

Gemellus superior

Obturator internus

Gemellus inferior

Pelvis

Obturator externus

Quadratus femoris

Femur

Deep six external rotators

The muscles in this group all originate from the pelvis and insert on the femur (thigh bone). They externally rotate the hip (or control internal rotation) and stabilize the sacroiliac joint during the loading and midstance phases of running (see pp.66–67). They maintain the alignment of the hip joint by keeping the ball centered in the socket during movement so that larger muscles can work effectively.

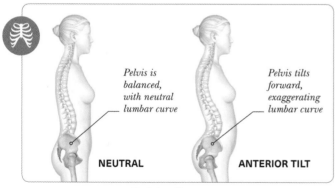

Pelvis is balanced, with neutral lumbar curve

Pelvis tilts forward, exaggerating lumbar curve

NEUTRAL

ANTERIOR TILT

Pelvic alignment

The degree of anterior pelvic tilt during running affects the amount of hip extension achieved in toe-off. While some anterior tilt is required, excessive tilt may increase the risk of femoroacetabular impingement (see p.27) and place the hip extensors at a mechanical disadvantage for generating force. To minimize excessive tilt, target the hip extensors with exercises and limit the time spent seated, which puts your hip flexors in a shortened position.

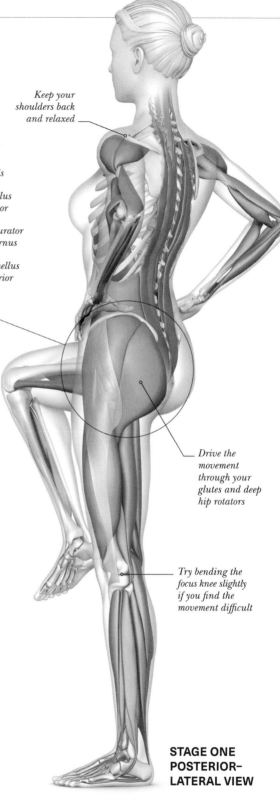

Keep your shoulders back and relaxed

Drive the movement through your glutes and deep hip rotators

Try bending the focus knee slightly if you find the movement difficult

STAGE ONE POSTERIOR-LATERAL VIEW

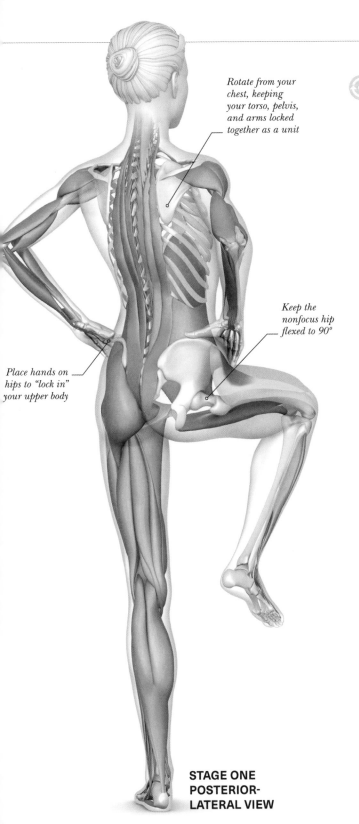

Rotate from your chest, keeping your torso, pelvis, and arms locked together as a unit

Keep the nonfocus hip flexed to 90°

Place hands on hips to "lock in" your upper body

STAGE ONE POSTERIOR-LATERAL VIEW

STANDING HIP ROTATION VARIATION
Supported Hip Rotation

If you have difficulty engaging your gluteal muscles while performing Standing Hip Rotation, wrap a resistance band around your knee to give your stance (focus) leg something to push against during the exercise.

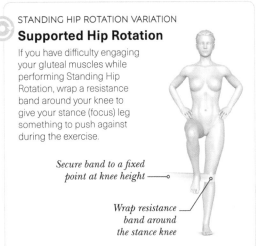

Secure band to a fixed point at knee height

Wrap resistance band around the stance knee

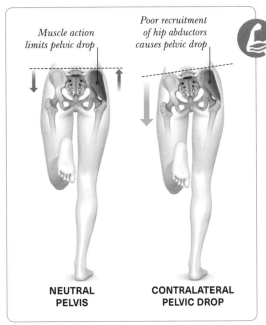

Muscle action limits pelvic drop

Poor recruitment of hip abductors causes pelvic drop

NEUTRAL PELVIS

CONTRALATERAL PELVIC DROP

Gluteus medius

This muscle is often referred to as a hip abductor, but rarely is this its function, as we almost never need to lift our thigh out to the side. (That is an "open-chain" action, with the foot not in contact with the ground.) Instead, the major function of the gluteus medius is its reverse action, when the foot is planted and the gluteus medius keeps the pelvis level. (This is a "closed-chain" action, with the foot connected to the ground.) In running, this function prevents excessive contralateral pelvic drop (see p.73) and excessive hip adduction during the loading phase of running.

129

HIP
EXTENSION

The gluteus maximus is the primary hip extensor and is an important contributor to the propulsion force in terminal stance (see p.68), especially as speeds increase. This exercise strengthens the gluteus maximus and reinforces its role as the primary hip extensor.

THE **BIG PICTURE**

You will need a resistance band for this exercise. Attach it to a secure point directly in front of you at ankle height. It should be taut enough to work the glutes and hamstrings as they extend the hip to draw the focus leg backward.

If new to the exercise, perform 3 sets of 15–20 reps on each side. To progress, increase the resistance by tightening the band or using a higher resistance band.

Hip and upper leg

As long as the movement during this stage is isolated to the hip, the **hip extensors**, including the **proximal glutes**, and the **proximal hamstrings** work concentrically to draw the leg back. Avoid arching and stretching through your lower back, so the work done to enable the movement remains at the hip. This can be a narrow range of movement, as hip extension is

Upper **body**

The **abdominal muscles** engage to maintain the neutral position of the pelvis and prevent it from tilting forward. Placing your hands on the crest of your pelvis allows you to monitor that movement and control the tilt.

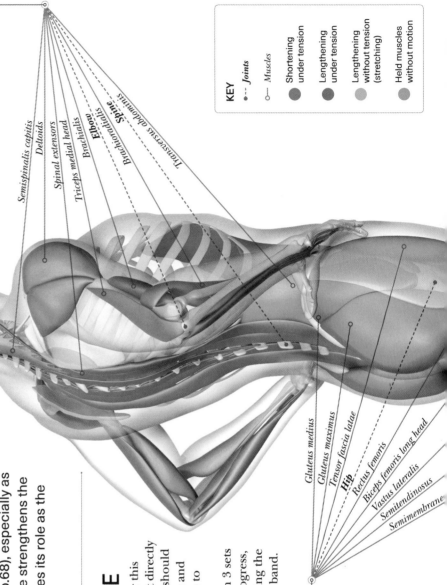

Semispinalis capitis
Deltoids
Spinal extensors
Triceps medial head
Brachialis
Elbow
Brachioradialis
Spine
Transversus abdominus

Gluteus medius
Gluteus maximus
Tensor fascia latae
Hip
Rectus femoris
Biceps femoris long head
Vastus lateralis
Semitendinosus
Semimembrane

KEY

--- *Joints*

o--- *Muscles*

● Shortening under tension

● Lengthening under tension

● Lengthening without tension (stretching)

● Held muscles without motion

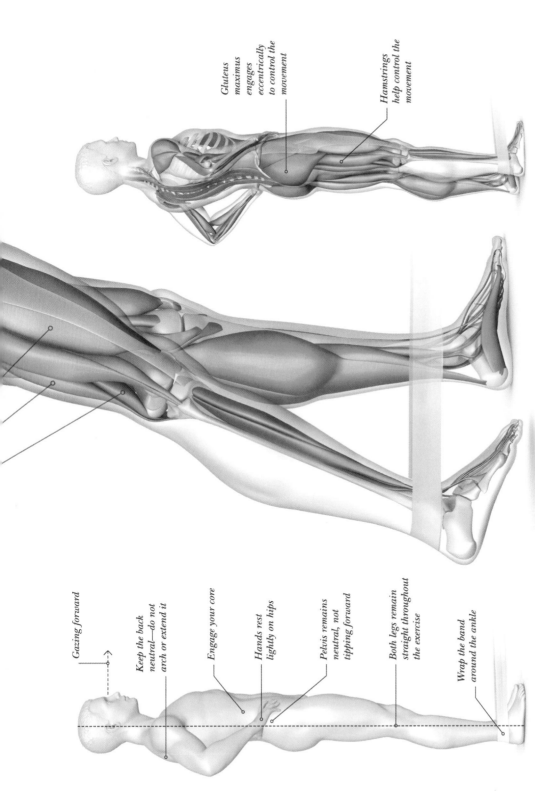

Gluteus maximus engages eccentrically to control the movement

Hamstrings help control the movement

STAGE TWO

As soon as your hip reaches the end of its range at the end of stage 1, immediately return it to the starting position in a slow, controlled movement. Repeat stages one and two.

STAGE ONE

Maintaining a neutral pelvis, use the gluteal muscles to slowly extend your hip, moving the focus heel backward. Take your leg only as far as your hip's range of motion allows. Do not arch your lower back or allow your pelvis to tilt forward.

Gazing forward

Keep the back neutral—do not arch or extend it

Engage your core

Hands rest lightly on hips

Pelvis remains neutral, not tipping forward

Both legs remain straight throughout the exercise

Wrap the band around the ankle

PREPARATORY STAGE

Reach down to wrap the resistance band around the ankle of the focus leg, then stand tall with your hands on your hips and your feet hip-distance apart.

TRADITIONAL
DEADLIFT

Building strength in the legs improves their capacity to absorb impact forces during the loading phase of the running cycle (see p.66) and also enhances performance in the propulsion phase (see p.68). This exercise strengthens the quadriceps, hamstrings, and glutes and can help protect you from running-related injuries.

THE BIG PICTURE

You will need a barbell for this exercise. The movement here is enabled by the hip and knee joints simultaneously extending, then flexing. Focus on the quads, hamstrings, and glutes to drive the upward movement.

If new to this exercise, perform 3 sets of 10–12 reps with light weight. To progress, increase the weight and reduce to 3 sets of 6–8 reps.

Caution

This exercise should be performed under the guidance of a physical therapist or certified strength trainer if you do not have experience with it.

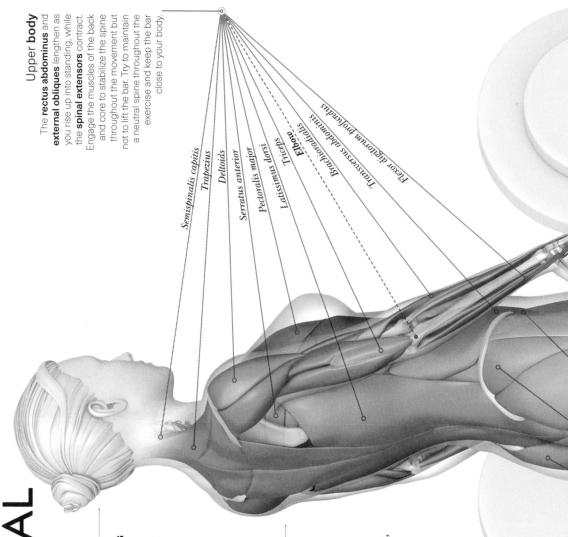

Upper **body**

The **rectus abdominus** and **external obliques** lengthen as you rise up into standing, while the **spinal extensors** contract. Engage the muscles of the back and core to stabilize the spine throughout the movement but not to lift the bar. Try to maintain a neutral spine throughout the exercise and keep the bar close to your body.

Semispinalis capitis

Trapezius

Deltoids

Serratus anterior

Pectoralis major

Latissimus dorsi

Triceps

Elbow

Brachioradialis

Transversus abdominis

Flexor digitorum profundus

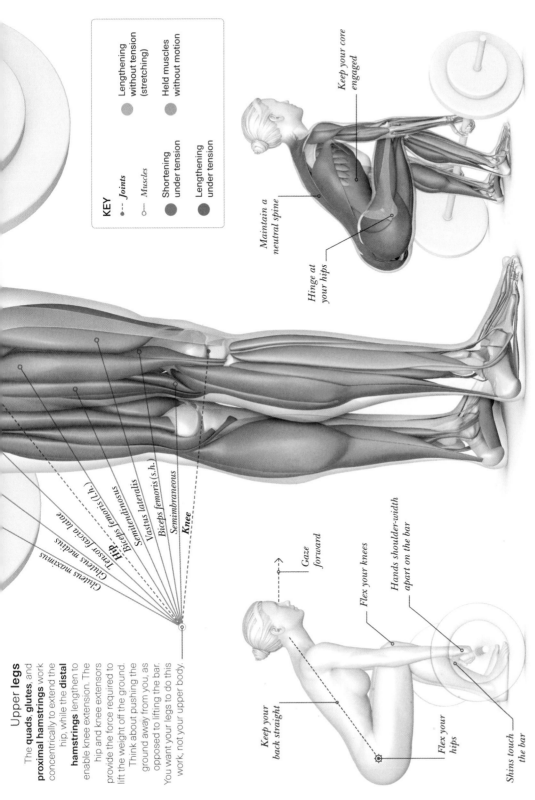

KEY

- – – – **Joints**
- ◦ **Muscles**
- ● Shortening under tension
- ● Lengthening under tension
- ● Lengthening without tension (stretching)
- ● Held muscles without motion

Upper legs

The **quads**, **glutes**, and **proximal hamstrings** work concentrically to extend the hip, while the **distal hamstrings** lengthen to enable knee extension. The hip and knee extensors provide the force required to lift the weight off the ground. Think about pushing the ground away from you, as opposed to lifting the bar. You want your legs to do this work, not your upper body.

Gluteus maximus
Gluteus medius
Tensor fascia latae
Hip
Biceps femoris (l.h.)
Semitendinosus
Vastus lateralis
Biceps femoris (s.h.)
Semimembraneous
Knee

Keep your core engaged

Maintain a neutral spine

Hinge at your hips

Gaze forward

Flex your knees

Hands shoulder-width apart on the bar

Keep your back straight

Flex your hips

Shins touch the bar

PREPARATORY STAGE

Stand with your feet hip-width apart and the bar over the center of your feet. Bend at your hips and knees to grip the bar. As you descend, your shins move toward the bar. When they touch it, stop descending. Squeeze your chest up to flatten your back and adopt a neutral spine position.

STAGE ONE

Take a deep breath in and, keeping your entire back and core engaged and your chest up, push through your heels and lift the barbell straight up, driving your hips forward as you lift. Hold at the top for 2 seconds.

STAGE TWO

Flexing your hips and knees, slowly (over 3 seconds) return the bar straight down to the floor. Repeat stages one and two.

» CLOSER LOOK

Traditional Deadlift is a simple exercise that delivers strength gains to the main lower-limb muscle groups. However, care should be taken to reduce strain on the lumbar spine (see p.30), especially for those who have recurrent lower back pain.

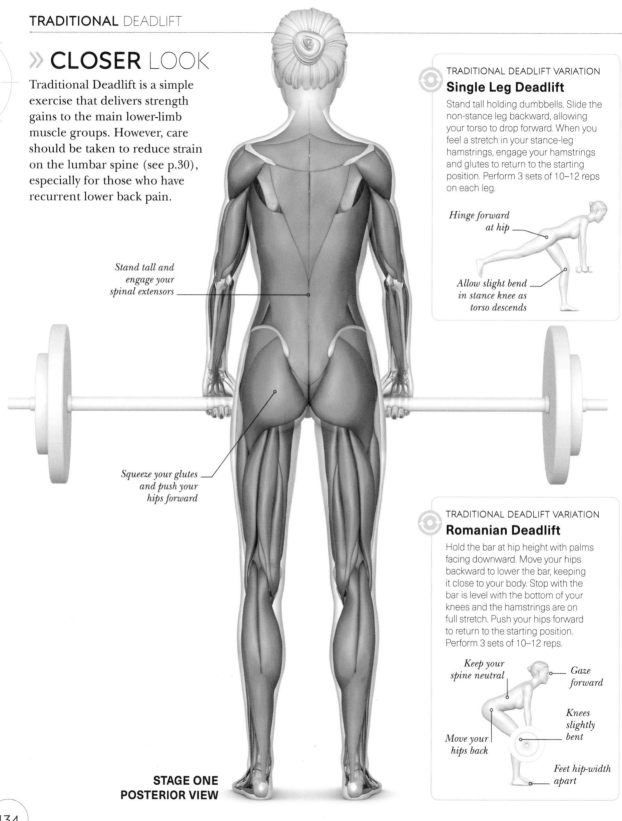

Stand tall and engage your spinal extensors

Squeeze your glutes and push your hips forward

**STAGE ONE
POSTERIOR VIEW**

TRADITIONAL DEADLIFT VARIATION
Single Leg Deadlift

Stand tall holding dumbbells. Slide the non-stance leg backward, allowing your torso to drop forward. When you feel a stretch in your stance-leg hamstrings, engage your hamstrings and glutes to return to the starting position. Perform 3 sets of 10–12 reps on each leg.

Hinge forward at hip

Allow slight bend in stance knee as torso descends

TRADITIONAL DEADLIFT VARIATION
Romanian Deadlift

Hold the bar at hip height with palms facing downward. Move your hips backward to lower the bar, keeping it close to your body. Stop with the bar is level with the bottom of your knees and the hamstrings are on full stretch. Push your hips forward to return to the starting position. Perform 3 sets of 10–12 reps.

Keep your spine neutral

Gaze forward

Knees slightly bent

Move your hips back

Feet hip-width apart

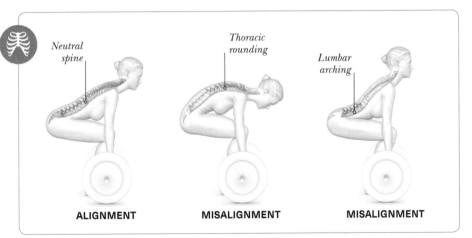

Neutral spine

Thoracic rounding

Lumbar arching

ALIGNMENT

MISALIGNMENT

MISALIGNMENT

Spinal **alignment**

When performing Traditional Deadlift, keep your spine in a neutral position, neither arching nor rounding it. Your hip muscles should bear the load. If you arch or round your back too much, not only do you reduce the load on the hip muscles, you also increase the risk of injuring your back.

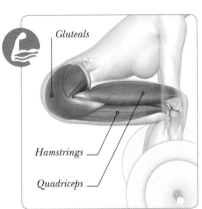

Gluteals

Hamstrings

Quadriceps

Developing **speed**

As running speed increases, power generation shifts from more distal musculature, such as the calf muscles, to proximal muscles like the glutes, quads, and hamstrings. To improve speed, build the capacity of these proximal muscle groups through targeted exercises like Traditional Deadlift.

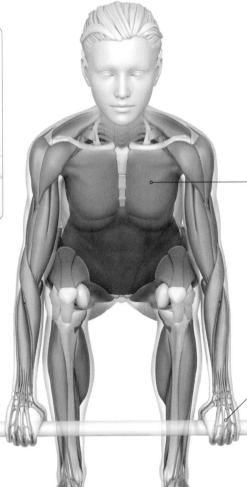

Engage your pectoral muscles to maintain a firm hold on the bar

If necessary, use chalk or wear gloves to keep a firm grip on the bar

STAGE TWO
ANTERIOR VIEW

SINGLE LEG
BALL SQUAT

Caution

If you experience anterior knee pain during this exercise, consult a physical therapist to ensure you are not aggravating your condition (see p.98).

The entire kinetic chain (see p.49) benefits from this exercise, which strengthens the core, hip, thigh, and calf muscles and also challenges your stability on one leg.

THE **BIG PICTURE**

You will need an exercise ball to perform this modified squat. Note that the stance leg should be slightly abducted throughout the exercise, making the gluteus medius work harder. Ensure the stance knee does not drop inward by aiming to maintain the knee's position in the sagittal plane (see p.10) as you move. Do not bend from the waist. Instead, drop straight down as you squat, keeping your torso upright and your hips level throughout.

If new to this exercise, aim for 3 sets of 5–10 reps on each side. Once you are able to maintain knee alignment, increase the weight (see p.99) and complete 3–4 sets of 6–8 reps.

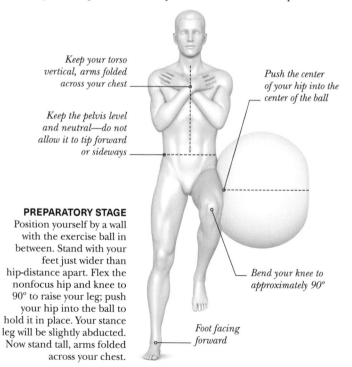

Keep your torso vertical, arms folded across your chest

Keep the pelvis level and neutral—do not allow it to tip forward or sideways

Push the center of your hip into the center of the ball

Bend your knee to approximately 90°

PREPARATORY STAGE

Position yourself by a wall with the exercise ball in between. Stand with your feet just wider than hip-distance apart. Flex the nonfocus hip and knee to 90° to raise your leg; push your hip into the ball to hold it in place. Your stance leg will be slightly abducted. Now stand tall, arms folded across your chest.

Foot facing forward

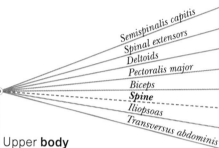

Semispinalis capitis
Spinal extensors
Deltoids
Pectoralis major
Biceps
Spine
Iliopsoas
Transversus abdominis

Upper body

The **abdominal muscles** engage to keep the body upright. Keep your hips level and your spine neutral, as if standing. Avoid rotating or bending sideways through your torso.

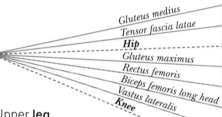

Gluteus medius
Tensor fascia latae
Hip
Gluteus maximus
Rectus femoris
Biceps femoris long head
Vastus lateralis
Knee

Upper leg

As you lower yourself by flexing your knee, the **glutes** and **quads** work eccentrically, which mimics the loading phase in running. The **hip abductors**, primarily the **gluteus medius**, have to work hard to maintain a level pelvis. Focus on the quads and glutes doing the main work.

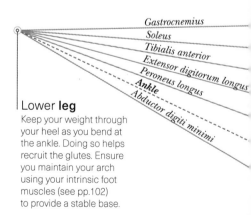

Gastrocnemius
Soleus
Tibialis anterior
Extensor digitorum longus
Peroneus longus
Ankle
Abductor digiti minimi

Lower leg

Keep your weight through your heel as you bend at the ankle. Doing so helps recruit the glutes. Ensure you maintain your arch using your intrinsic foot muscles (see pp.102) to provide a stable base.

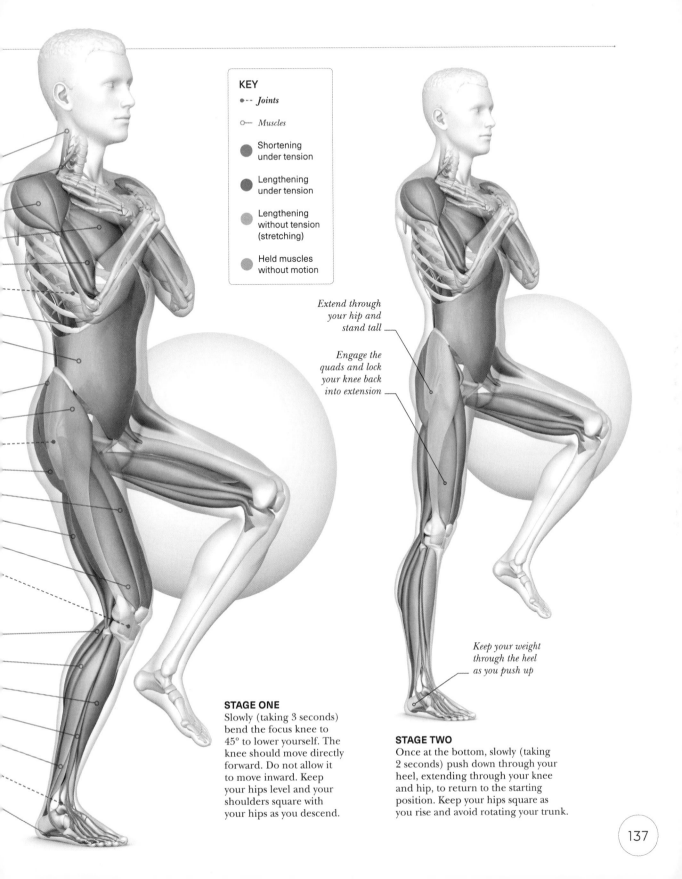

KEY

●-- *Joints*

○— *Muscles*

● Shortening under tension

● Lengthening under tension

● Lengthening without tension (stretching)

● Held muscles without motion

Extend through your hip and stand tall

Engage the quads and lock your knee back into extension

Keep your weight through the heel as you push up

STAGE ONE
Slowly (taking 3 seconds) bend the focus knee to 45° to lower yourself. The knee should move directly forward. Do not allow it to move inward. Keep your hips level and your shoulders square with your hips as you descend.

STAGE TWO
Once at the bottom, slowly (taking 2 seconds) push down through your heel, extending through your knee and hip, to return to the starting position. Keep your hips square as you rise and avoid rotating your trunk.

» CLOSER LOOK

This dynamic exercise challenges the core and hips. By adding a rotation at the pelvis or chest (see opposite), the movements of the exercise mimic how the body engages the diagonal elastic support mechanism (see p.49) during the running motion.

Core strength

The core needs strength to control the upper body as it passes over the supporting leg during the stance phase of running (see pp.66–68), as well as to stabilize the pelvis, which provides the upper leg muscles a sturdy base from which to generate propulsive power. The core also negotiates substantial forces being transferred through it from both above and below. Single Leg Ball Squat develops the muscles of the core, as well as the upper leg.

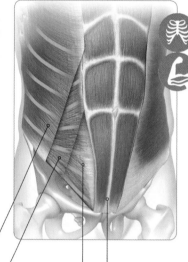

External obliques

Internal obliques

Transversus abdominus

Rectus abdominus

Keep your shoulders level

Engage your core muscles to maintain a neutral spine and pelvis

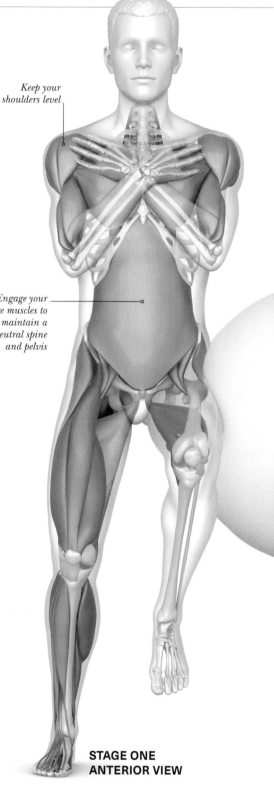

STAGE ONE ANTERIOR VIEW

SINGLE LEG SQUAT VARIATION

Targeting the quads

If you want to increase the demand on the quads and reduce that on the glutes while performing Single Leg Ball Squat, place a heel wedge under your heel to shift your weight onto your forefoot. This variation may be of help if rehabilitating from patellar tendinopathy.

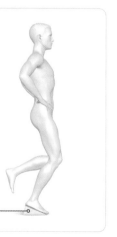

Place wedge under heel

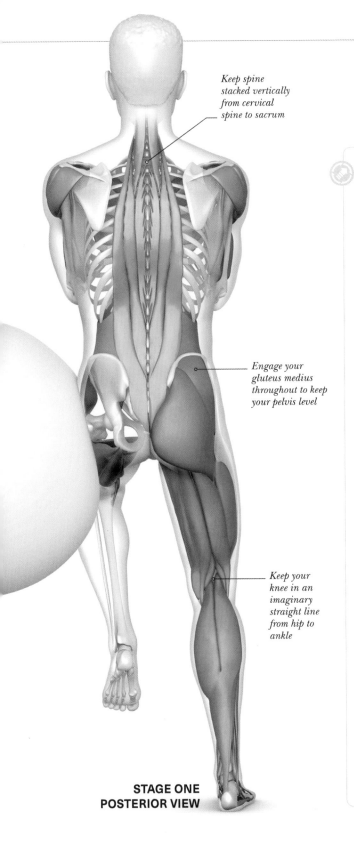

Keep spine stacked vertically from cervical spine to sacrum

Engage your gluteus medius throughout to keep your pelvis level

Keep your knee in an imaginary straight line from hip to ankle

STAGE ONE POSTERIOR VIEW

SINGLE LEG SQUAT PROGRESSIONS

Adding chest or pelvic rotation

When performing the Single Leg Ball Squat, add rotation of either your pelvis or chest each time you are in the squat. Rotate to one side, then the other, in a smooth, flowing movement before pushing back up. When rotating your chest, keep your hips square so that you rotate only the thoracic spine (see p.30). If rotating your pelvis, keep your chest square and facing forward so that you move only your hips.

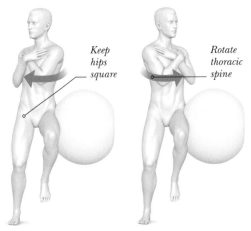

Keep hips square

Rotate thoracic spine

CHEST ROTATION

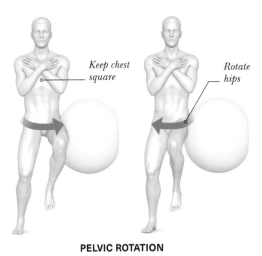

Keep chest square

Rotate hips

PELVIC ROTATION

HAMSTRING
BALL ROLL-IN

This exercise strengthens the hamstrings and core, and can be used to aid in recovery from hamstring strains and other running-related injuries (see pp.54–63). The hamstrings play an important role in running performance, especially speed.

THE **BIG PICTURE**

You will need an exercise ball with a diameter of 21½–26 in (55–65 cm) for this exercise. This is a challenging maneuver. Once you have raised your body and positioned it in a straight line at the start of the exercise, focus on maintaining the position of your trunk and hips throughout the movement. Much of the work here is in preventing your hips from descending as you roll the ball in and out.

If you are new to this exercise, perform 3 sets of 10–12 reps. Once you can hold the position of your hips and torso throughout the exercise, remove the support of your forearms (cross them over your chest). To progress, perform this as a single-leg exercise. Flex the knee of the nonfocus leg and bring it toward your chest to keep the leg out of the way when the focus leg rolls the ball in.

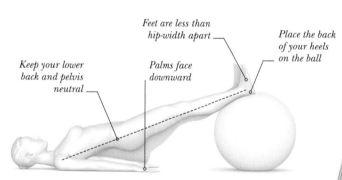

Keep your lower back and pelvis neutral

Feet are less than hip-width apart

Palms face downward

Place the back of your heels on the ball

PREPARATORY STAGE
Lie on your back with your arms by your sides. Rest your heels close together on the exercise ball. Now raise your hips so that your body forms a straight line from your shoulder through your hip and knee to your ankle. Keep your spine in a neutral position.

Upper **leg**
The **hamstrings** produce the knee flexion in this stage. Dig your heels into the ball and focus on pulling it in toward you, rather than raising your knees. The **glutes** engage to maintain the bridging action that keeps your hips raised, and lengthen as your hip flexes. The **hip flexors** in the front of your hip engage concentrically to flex your hip.

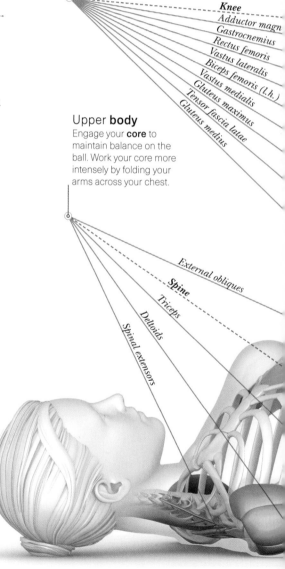

Knee
Adductor magn.
Gastrocnemius
Rectus femoris
Vastus lateralis
Biceps femoris (l.h.)
Vastus medialis
Gluteus maximus
Tensor fascia latae
Gluteus medius

Upper **body**
Engage your **core** to maintain balance on the ball. Work your core more intensely by folding your arms across your chest.

External obliques
Spine
Triceps
Deltoids
Spinal extensors

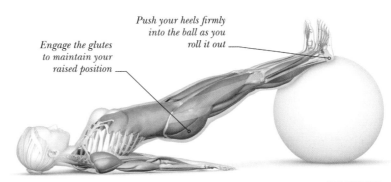

KEY

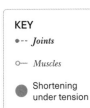

- •-- *Joints*
- o— *Muscles*
- Shortening under tension
- Lengthening under tension
- Lengthening without tension (stretching)
- Held muscles without motion

Engage the glutes to maintain your raised position

Push your heels firmly into the ball as you roll it out

STAGE TWO
Slowly roll the ball back to the starting position while keeping your hips raised. When your legs are fully extended, hold the position for a moment, then repeat stages one and two.

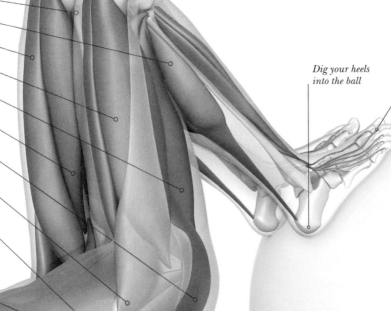

Dig your heels into the ball

Relax your toes

Keep your back raised as you roll the ball in

STAGE ONE
Flex your hip and knee to slowly roll the ball toward you while keeping your hips raised off the floor. Hold for 2 seconds.

LUNGE

The Lunge is a great exercise to target strength in both lower limbs in a running-specific pose. It works the muscles both eccentrically and concentrically.

THE BIG PICTURE

Although both legs are working hard in this exercise, it is the glutes and quads of the front leg that are targeted. As you lunge, move downward, not forward. When in the lunge, your shoulder, hip, and (lowered) back knee should be aligned vertically. Throughout the exercise, ensure your weight is evenly distributed through your flat front foot and the dorsiflexed toes of your back foot. Your arms move in running motion in coordination with your leg movements. As you lunge, raise the arm on the opposite side of your body to the front leg. Reverse the arm movement as you rise out of the lunge.

If new to this exercise, perform 3 sets of 8–12 reps on each side. To increase the load on the glutes of the front leg, hold a dumbbell on the opposite side of the body to the front leg.

Upper **body**
By mimicking the running motion, the muscles of the **arms** and **torso** engage to counterbalance the movement in the lower limbs.

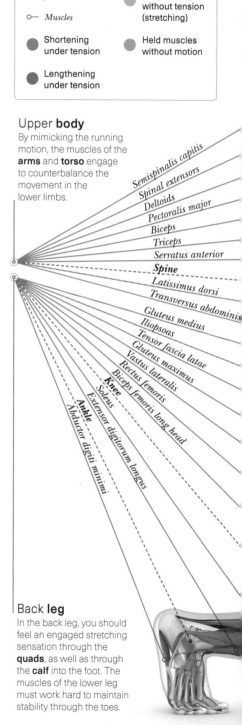

Semispinalis capitis
Spinal extensors
Deltoids
Pectoralis major
Biceps
Triceps
Serratus anterior
Spine
Latissimus dorsi
Transversus abdominis
Gluteus medius
Iliopsoas
Tensor fascia latae
Gluteus maximus
Vastus lateralis
Rectus femoris
Knee
Biceps femoris long head
Ankle
Soleus
Extensor digitorum longus
Abductor digiti minimi

> **! Caution**
> If you have anterior knee pain during this exercise, consult a physical therapist to ensure you are not aggravating your condition (see p.98).

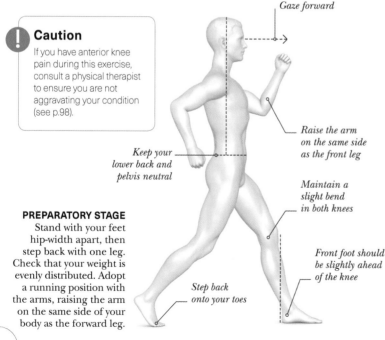

Gaze forward

Raise the arm on the same side as the front leg

Keep your lower back and pelvis neutral

Maintain a slight bend in both knees

Front foot should be slightly ahead of the knee

Step back onto your toes

PREPARATORY STAGE
Stand with your feet hip-width apart, then step back with one leg. Check that your weight is evenly distributed. Adopt a running position with the arms, raising the arm on the same side of your body as the forward leg.

Back **leg**
In the back leg, you should feel an engaged stretching sensation through the **quads**, as well as through the **calf** into the foot. The muscles of the lower leg must work hard to maintain stability through the toes.

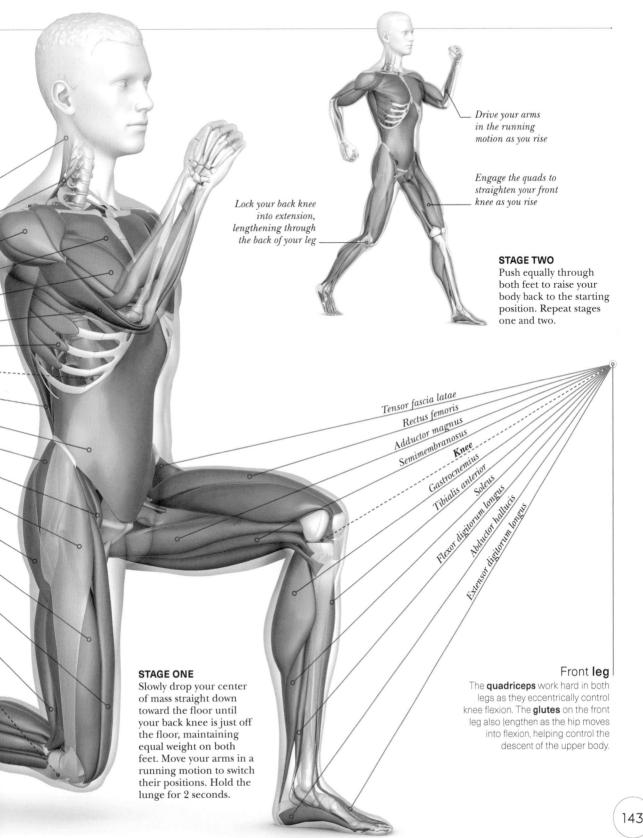

Drive your arms in the running motion as you rise

Engage the quads to straighten your front knee as you rise

Lock your back knee into extension, lengthening through the back of your leg

STAGE TWO
Push equally through both feet to raise your body back to the starting position. Repeat stages one and two.

Tensor fascia latae
Rectus femoris
Adductor magnus
Semimembranosus
Knee
Gastrocnemius
Tibialis anterior
Soleus
Flexor digitorum longus
Abductor hallucis
Extensor digitorum longus

STAGE ONE
Slowly drop your center of mass straight down toward the floor until your back knee is just off the floor, maintaining equal weight on both feet. Move your arms in a running motion to switch their positions. Hold the lunge for 2 seconds.

Front **leg**
The **quadriceps** work hard in both legs as they eccentrically control knee flexion. The **glutes** on the front leg also lengthen as the hip moves into flexion, helping control the descent of the upper body.

143

FRONT PLANK
WITH ROTATION

Also known as "mountain climber," this exercise strengthens the muscles of the core, especially the oblique muscles. It also improves the efficiency of the diagonal elastic support mechanism (see p.49), which enables the transfer of forces between the lower and upper body while running.

Feet are slightly apart

Body forms a straight line

Dorsiflexed toes bear weight

Elbows align with shoulders vertically

PREPARATORY STAGE
Lie on your front with your upper body propped up on your forearms. To get into starting position, lift your hips off the floor so that your body forms a straight line from your head though your navel to your ankle.

THE **BIG PICTURE**

Mountain Climber improves balance and coordination, as well as core strength. Once you have raised your hips into the starting position, bring your body into a straight line from head to ankle, then focus on maintaining this line as you work your legs. Use your core muscles to prevent your back from dipping toward the floor as you move.

Perform 3 sets of 10–15 reps. To progress, increase the number of repetitions.

KEY
- •-- *Joints*
- ○— *Muscles*
- ● Shortening under tension
- ● Lengthening under tension
- ● Lengthening without tension (stretching)
- ● Held muscles without motion

Leg
Initiate the movement from your hips, engaging the **hip flexors** to drive your knee up and out to the opposite side. Your knee flexes to 90°. The **quads** in the opposite leg engage to support your weight.

Gastrocnemius

Knee

Vastus lateralis

Rectus femoris

Vastus medialis

Tensor fascia latae

⚠ Caution
If you have lower back pain while performing this exercise, consult a physical therapist to ensure you are not aggravating your condition (see p.98).

Core and arms

The obliques drive the movement of your leg across your body, producing a rotation in your pelvis. The **external obliques** work concentrically on the side of your supporting leg and eccentrically on the other side. The arms engage to hold and stabilize your position. The **spinal extensors** in your lower back hold your spine in a neutral position to avoid excessive arching.

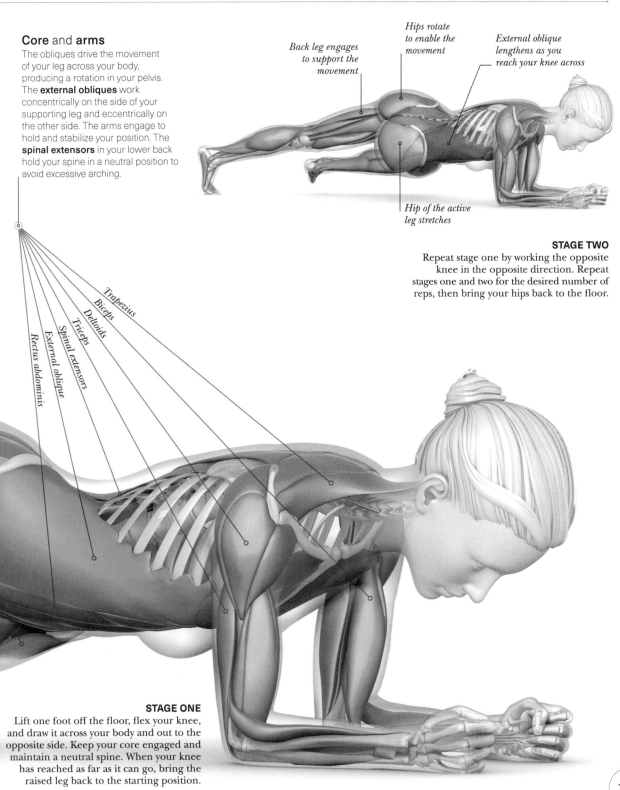

Back leg engages to support the movement

Hips rotate to enable the movement

External oblique lengthens as you reach your knee across

Hip of the active leg stretches

STAGE TWO
Repeat stage one by working the opposite knee in the opposite direction. Repeat stages one and two for the desired number of reps, then bring your hips back to the floor.

Trapezius
Biceps
Deltoids
Triceps
Spinal extensors
External oblique
Rectus abdominis

STAGE ONE
Lift one foot off the floor, flex your knee, and draw it across your body and out to the opposite side. Keep your core engaged and maintain a neutral spine. When your knee has reached as far as it can go, bring the raised leg back to the starting position.

» CLOSER LOOK

Front Plank with Rotation is an alternative to the static plank exercise and requires controlled rotation through your core while maintaining spinal stability. Ensure you focus the movement to the areas of your spine that produce rotation and not through the lumbar spine (see p.30).

Generating power in the upper body

It is important for runners to include in their drills exercises that target their upper body. As you run, you generate power with with your upper and lower body, especially at greater speeds. Rotation of the torso can help drive the lower limbs in the sagittal plane (see p.10) via the diagonal elastic support mechanism (see p.49). Alternating paired contractions of the external obliques and their opposite internal obliques helps drive this rotation.

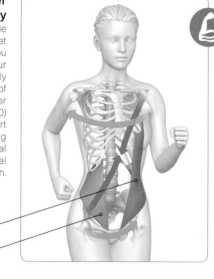

External obliques ——

Internal obliques ——

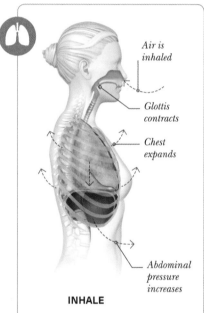

Air is inhaled

— *Glottis contracts*

— *Chest expands*

— *Abdominal pressure increases*

INHALE

Keep breathing!

It is easy to stiffen your abdominal muscles and hold your breath when performing Front Plank with Rotation, but it is important to keep breathing evenly and regularly. When you hold your breath, you increase the intra-abdominal pressure, which stiffens your spine and reduces your ability to rotate. Instead, try to breathe freely throughout the movement as you would if you were running.

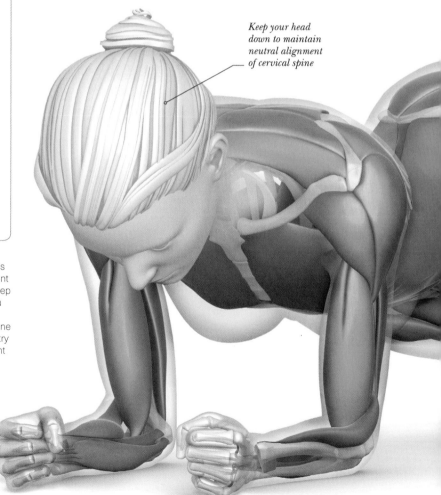

Keep your head down to maintain neutral alignment of cervical spine

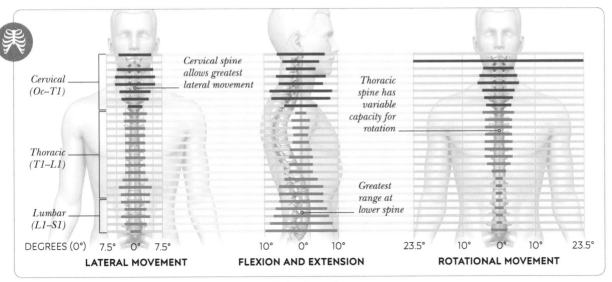

Cervical
(Oc–T1)

Cervical spine allows greatest lateral movement

Thoracic spine has variable capacity for rotation

Thoracic
(T1–L1)

Lumbar
(L1–S1)

Greatest range at lower spine

DEGREES (0°)   7.5°   0°   7.5° | 10°   0°   10° | 23.5°   10°   0°   10°   23.5°

LATERAL MOVEMENT   **FLEXION AND EXTENSION**   **ROTATIONAL MOVEMENT**

Spinal motion

In Front Plank with Rotation, the rotation is through the thorax, not the lower back. Different segments of your spine allow for specific movements (see p.30) through the three planes of motion. During running, upper body rotation should occur predominantly through the thoracic region, with the head and neck held still. The lumbar spine should contribute a small amount to flexion and extension as a result of movement of the pelvis in the sagittal plane.

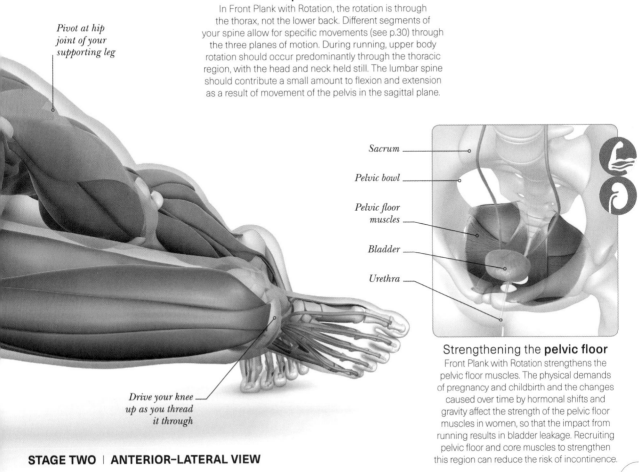

Pivot at hip joint of your supporting leg

Sacrum

Pelvic bowl

Pelvic floor muscles

Bladder

Urethra

Drive your knee up as you thread it through

STAGE TWO | ANTERIOR-LATERAL VIEW

Strengthening the **pelvic floor**

Front Plank with Rotation strengthens the pelvic floor muscles. The physical demands of pregnancy and childbirth and the changes caused over time by hormonal shifts and gravity affect the strength of the pelvic floor muscles in women, so that the impact from running results in bladder leakage. Recruiting pelvic floor and core muscles to strengthen this region can reduce the risk of incontinence.

SIDE PLANK
WITH ROTATION

> ⓘ **Caution**
> If you feel lower back pain during this exercise, consult a physical therapist to ensure you are not aggravating your condition (see p.98).

This exercise strengthens the core and can improve the efficiency of the diagonal elastic support mechanism (see p.49). The alternating rotational movements teach you to dissociate the chest and pelvis, which helps when running.

Hips
The **hip adductors** in the top leg, along with the **hip abductors** on the bottom leg, engage to keep your body off the ground and maintain a neutral posture at the hips and spine.

THE **BIG PICTURE**

In this exercise, all the action takes place between the thoracic spine (see p.30) and your thighs. Your knees and chest stay facing forward throughout, and everything between them rotates. As your hips turn, do not turn your chest and rotate your torso.

Perform 3 sets of 10–15 reps on each side, moving between the stages in a smooth, continuous movement.

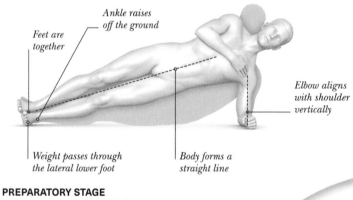

Ankle raises off the ground

Feet are together

Elbow aligns with shoulder vertically

Weight passes through the lateral lower foot

Body forms a straight line

Tensor fascia latae
Hip
Gluteus maximus
Gluteus medius
Iliopsoas
Adductor magnus

PREPARATORY STAGE
Lie down on one side with feet together and upper body propped up on your forearm. Fold the other arm across your chest. Raise your hips off the floor so your body forms a straight line.

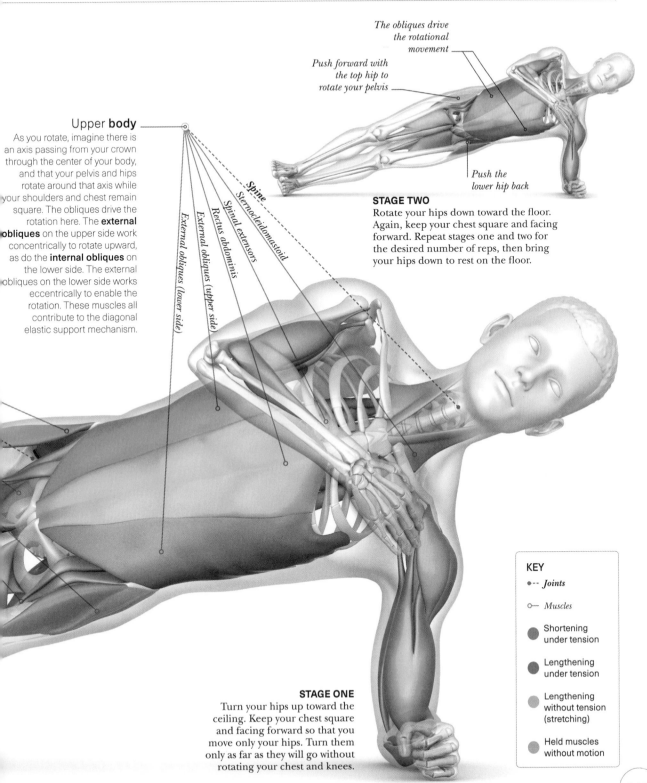

Upper body

As you rotate, imagine there is an axis passing from your crown through the center of your body, and that your pelvis and hips rotate around that axis while your shoulders and chest remain square. The obliques drive the rotation here. The **external obliques** on the upper side work concentrically to rotate upward, as do the **internal obliques** on the lower side. The external obliques on the lower side works eccentrically to enable the rotation. These muscles all contribute to the diagonal elastic support mechanism.

The obliques drive the rotational movement

Push forward with the top hip to rotate your pelvis

Push the lower hip back

STAGE TWO

Rotate your hips down toward the floor. Again, keep your chest square and facing forward. Repeat stages one and two for the desired number of reps, then bring your hips down to rest on the floor.

Spine

Sternocleidomastoid

Spinal extensors

Rectus abdominis

External obliques (upper side)

External obliques (lower side)

STAGE ONE

Turn your hips up toward the ceiling. Keep your chest square and facing forward so that you move only your hips. Turn them only as far as they will go without rotating your chest and knees.

KEY

•-- *Joints*

○— *Muscles*

● Shortening under tension

● Lengthening under tension

● Lengthening without tension (stretching)

● Held muscles without motion

BOX JUMP

Box Jump improves the stiffness of the leg springs
(see p.98) and aids in the energy storage and release
capacity of the glutes, quads, calves, and hip abductors.
This improves control of knee and hip alignment
during the loading phase of running (see p.66),
aiding in performance, as well as injury prevention.

THE **BIG PICTURE**

You will need a box for this exercise. Select a 12-in
(30-cm) high box if new to jumping drills. Bend
your knees to roughly 45° for take-off and landing.

Perform 3 sets of 10–12 reps. To progress,
increase the height of the box and reduce to
3–4 sets of 6–8 reps.

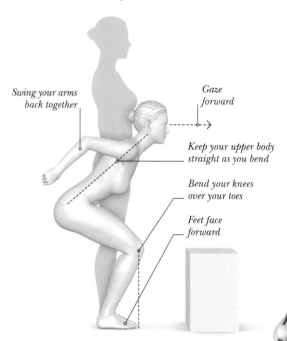

*Swing your arms
back together*

*Gaze
forward*

*Keep your upper body
straight as you bend*

*Bend your knees
over your toes*

*Feet face
forward*

STAGE ONE
Stand tall with the box in front of you,
with feet hip-width apart and arms by
your sides. Now bend your knees, ready
to spring. Raise your elbows behind you,
preparing to swing your arms forward.

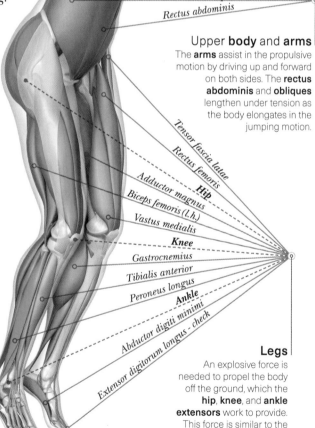

STAGE TWO
Forcefully drive up
through your legs,
extending at your
ankle, knee, and hip,
to jump up and forward
onto the box. At the
same time, drive your
arms forward and up.

Biceps
Triceps
Deltoids
Pectoralis major
Latissimus dorsi
Serratus anterior
External oblique
Rectus abdominis

Upper **body** and **arms**
The **arms** assist in the propulsive
motion by driving up and forward
on both sides. The **rectus
abdominis** and **obliques**
lengthen under tension as
the body elongates in the
jumping motion.

Tensor fascia latae
Rectus femoris
Hip
Adductor magnus
Biceps femoris (l.h.)
Vastus medialis
Knee
Gastrocnemius
Tibialis anterior
Peroneus longus
Ankle
Abductor digiti minimi
Extensor digitorum longus - check

Legs
An explosive force is
needed to propel the body
off the ground, which the
hip, **knee**, and **ankle
extensors** work to provide.
This force is similar to the
propulsion forces generated
during terminal stance in
running (see p.68).

150

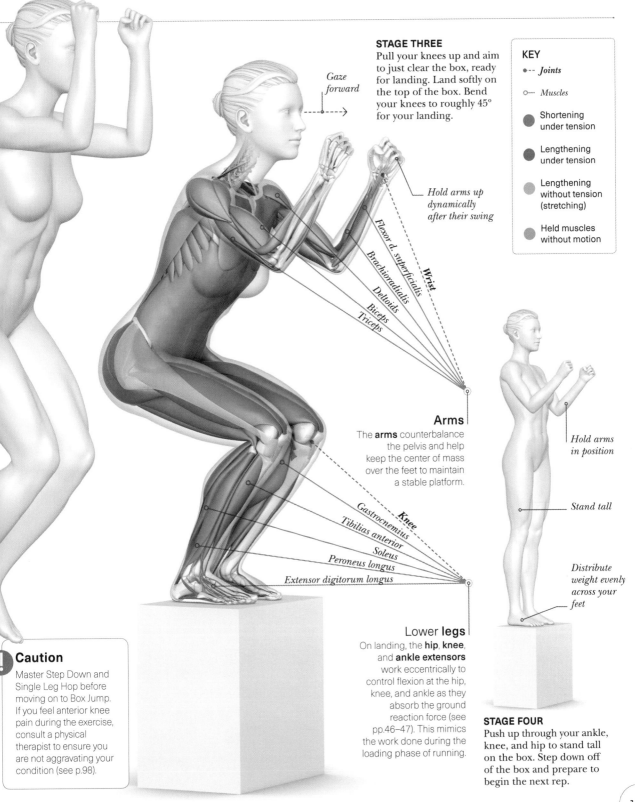

STAGE THREE
Pull your knees up and aim to just clear the box, ready for landing. Land softly on the top of the box. Bend your knees to roughly 45° for your landing.

Gaze forward

Hold arms up dynamically after their swing

Flexor d. superficialis
Brachioradialis
Deltoids
Biceps
Triceps

Wrist

KEY
- •--- *Joints*
- ○— *Muscles*
- ● Shortening under tension
- ● Lengthening under tension
- ● Lengthening without tension (stretching)
- ● Held muscles without motion

Arms
The **arms** counterbalance the pelvis and help keep the center of mass over the feet to maintain a stable platform.

Knee

Gastrocnemius
Tibilias anterior
Soleus
Peroneus longus
Extensor digitorum longus

Lower **legs**
On landing, the **hip, knee**, and **ankle extensors** work eccentrically to control flexion at the hip, knee, and ankle as they absorb the ground reaction force (see pp.46–47). This mimics the work done during the loading phase of running.

Hold arms in position

Stand tall

Distribute weight evenly across your feet

STAGE FOUR
Push up through your ankle, knee, and hip to stand tall on the box. Step down off of the box and prepare to begin the next rep.

! Caution
Master Step Down and Single Leg Hop before moving on to Box Jump. If you feel anterior knee pain during the exercise, consult a physical therapist to ensure you are not aggravating your condition (see p.98).

151

» CLOSER LOOK

Box Jump is an advanced exercise that develops power through the lower-limb extensor muscles while also demanding control when landing to avoid high impacts. The high loads developed help make the bones stronger and less vulnerable to stress injuries caused by the repetitive load in running. Box jumps also expose the lower-limb muscles to greater forces, which can build capacity in these muscles beyond what can be achieved with running alone. As with the main exercise, the variations shown here are advanced exercises, so the same cautions apply (see p.151).

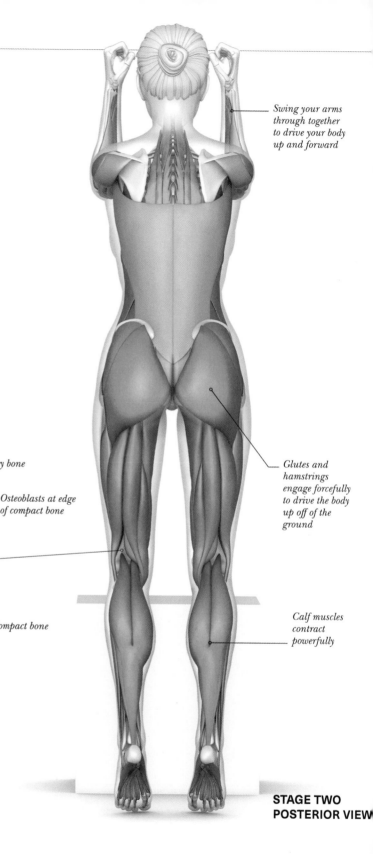

Swing your arms through together to drive your body up and forward

Glutes and hamstrings engage forcefully to drive the body up off of the ground

Calf muscles contract powerfully

STAGE TWO POSTERIOR VIEW

Osteon

Spongy bone

Osteoblasts at edge of compact bone

Compact bone

Strengthening the **bones**

Bones, like other tissues in the body, increase in strength in response to loading. However, studies have shown that long-distance running does not decrease the risk for stress fracture, because the cyclical low-strain nature of running is not sufficient to induce bone strengthening. Exercises that rapidly subject the body to high loads, such as hopping or jumping off of a box (see opposite), are recommended to stiffen bone and reduce stress fracture risk.

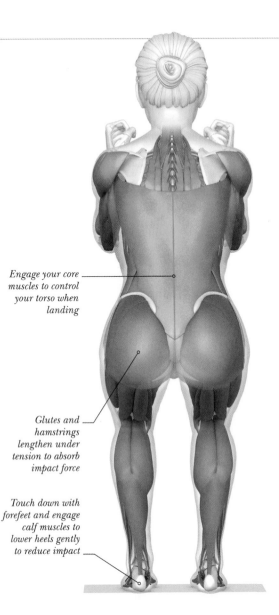

Engage your core muscles to control your torso when landing

Glutes and hamstrings lengthen under tension to absorb impact force

Touch down with forefeet and engage calf muscles to lower heels gently to reduce impact

STAGE THREE | POSTERIOR VIEW

BOX JUMP PROGRESSION

Single Leg Box Jump

Stand tall behind the box. Shift your weight onto the focus leg and bend your other knee to 90°. Maintaining a level pelvis, slowly bend the focus knee to approximately 45°, then forcefully drive up, extending at your ankle, knee, and hip, hopping up and forward onto the box. Land on the box and push up through your ankle, knee, and hip to stand tall. Step down off of the box. Use a 12-in (30-cm) high box and perform 3 sets of 10–12 reps. To progress, use a higher box and reduce to 3–4 sets of 6–8 reps.

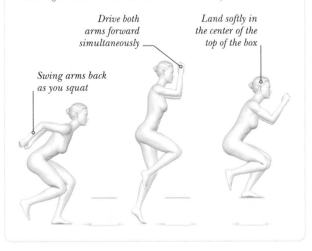

Drive both arms forward simultaneously

Land softly in the center of the top of the box

Swing arms back as you squat

BOX JUMP VARIATION

Jumping off of the box

Box Jump focuses on the propulsive phase of running (see p.68). Reverse it to mimic the demands of the loading phase (see p.66). Stand tall on the box. Bend your knees and hips, then jump up off the box and land softly and quietly, bending into a squat. Perform 3 sets of 10–12 reps. To progress the exercise, add weight (see p.99) and reduce to 3 sets of 6–8 reps, then move on to performing on one leg.

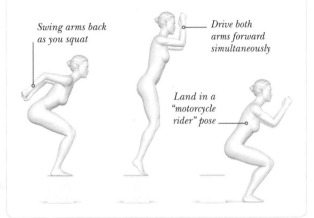

Swing arms back as you squat

Drive both arms forward simultaneously

Land in a "motorcycle rider" pose

SINGLE LEG HOP

Hopping on one leg is a great way to strengthen the glutes, quads, calves, and Achilles tendon. These muscles are essential in controlling knee and hip alignment during the loading phase of running (see p.66). This exercise increases the energy storage and release capacity of these muscles and improves the stiffness of the leg springs.

THE BIG PICTURE

Place a target on the floor for this exercise. (Try taping a cross to the floor.) Focus on the position of the stance-leg knee as you prepare to hop, and do not allow it to buckle inward. Maintain its position in the frontal plane (see p.10) as you squat. Bend your knee to roughly 45° for take-off and landing. Keep your pelvis level throughout the jump, and do not allow it to tilt forward.

If new to this exercise, perform 3 sets of 30-second reps on each side. To progress, increase the weight and/or the hopping time. Then progress to Box Jump (see pp.150–151).

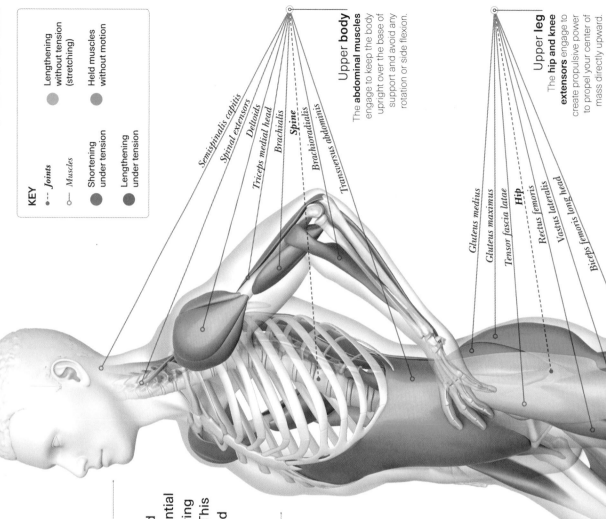

KEY

- - - *Joints*

○— *Muscles*

● Shortening under tension

● Lengthening under tension

● Lengthening without tension (stretching)

● Held muscles without motion

Semispinalis capitis

Spinal extensors

Deltoids

Triceps medial head

Brachialis

Spine

Brachioradialis

Transversus abdominis

Upper **body**

The **abdominal muscles** engage to keep the body upright over the base of support and avoid any rotation or side flexion.

Gluteus medius

Gluteus maximus

Tensor fascia latae

Hip

Rectus femoris

Vastus lateralis

Biceps femoris long head

Upper **leg**

The **hip and knee extensors** engage to create propulsive power to propel your center of mass directly upward.

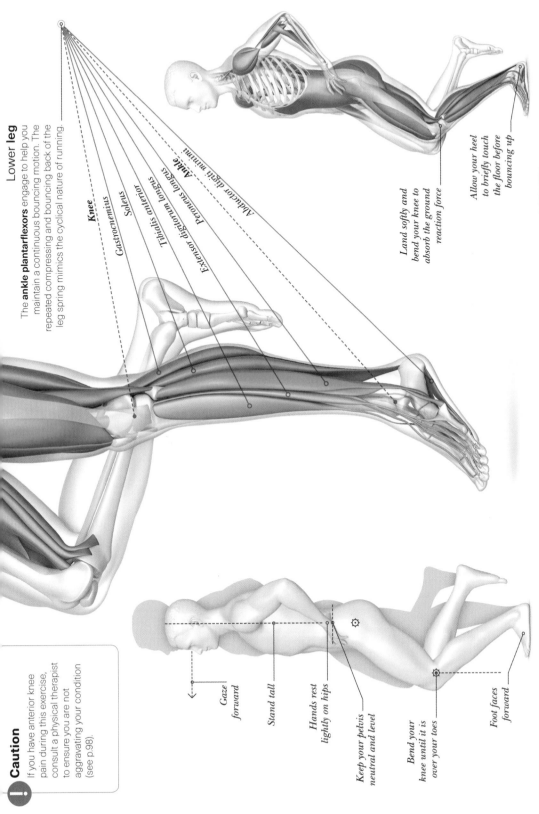

Lower leg

The **ankle plantarflexors** engage to help you maintain a continuous bouncing motion. The repeated compressing and bouncing back of the leg spring mimics the cyclical nature of running.

Knee

Gastrocnemius

Soleus

Tibialis anterior

Peroneus longus

Extensor digitorum longus

Ankle

Abductor digiti minimi

Land softly and bend your knee to absorb the ground reaction force

Allow your heel to briefly touch the floor before bouncing up

LANDING

Aim to land on the middle of the target, bending your knee to roughly 45° as you absorb the impact forces through your ankle, knee, and hip. Push straight up into the next hop. Aim to minimize the time spent on the ground.

TAKE-OFF

Forcefully push up through the focus leg, extending at your ankle, knee, and hip to hop straight up into the air.

PREPARATORY STAGE

Stand tall with the foot of the focus leg on the target and hands on hips. Shift your weight into the focus leg, then bend your other knee to 90° and raise your foot off the floor. Maintaining a level pelvis, slowly bend the focus-leg knee to roughly 45°.

Gaze forward

Stand tall

Hands rest lightly on hips

Keep your pelvis neutral and level

Bend your knee until it is over your toes

Foot faces forward

! Caution

If you have anterior knee pain during this exercise, consult a physical therapist to ensure you are not aggravating your condition (see p.98).

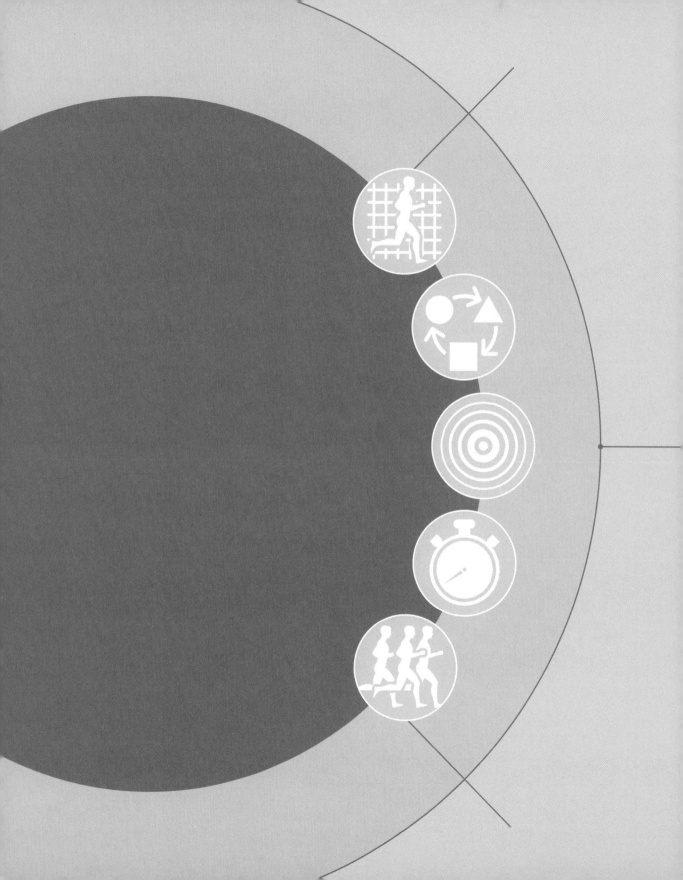

HOW TO TRAIN

Training smarter by targeting individual strengths and needs can take you to new levels of performance. In this chapter, we provide all the information you need to make your training show—and keep showing—solid results. We share tools to help you draw up bespoke training plans and provide a range of programs that can guide you, session by session, from your couch all the way to advanced marathoning.

WHY TRAIN?

The simplicity of running is one its greatest pleasures. You can pull on a pair of running shoes, head out the door, and just go. However, using a structured, goal-orientated training plan can improve performance, reduce injury risk, and make running even more enjoyable. It is worth considering the benefits.

AVOID INJURY

Because most running-related injuries result from overtraining, planning your workouts is a key factor in preventing injury. A training plan not only allows you to schedule the intensity of your workouts, it also helps you build in adequate time for recovery after long or hard runs. Incorporating easy days or weeks into your schedule will help your body adapt to the stresses of training and reduce the likelihood of getting injured. The drills, warm-ups, and stretches that are part of a structured workout also help prevent injury.

PERSONALIZE

Structuring and planning your training allows you to discover what works for you as an individual. When you follow a training program, you will have a record of the workouts you have done, which makes it easier to look back at what worked well for you and what did not. You can use this knowledge to make suitable adjustments to your training programs in the future.

IMPROVE
YOUR FORM

Consciously practicing your running form (see pp.74–75) will bring improvements and help you maintain good form even when running at a fast pace or if fatigued. When practiced with drills (see pp.84–89), your form becomes more natural and relaxed, which leads to better running economy (see p.165). Additionally, as you become fitter through structured training, your body makes beneficial adaptations that increase your lactate threshold, your VO_2 max, and endurance.

BENEFITS
OF TRAINING

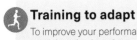 ## Training to adapt

To improve your performance, a training plan introduces workouts of increasing intensity. This places your body under the stress it needs to promote physical adaptations such as increased lactate threshold and VO_2 max (see p.37). However, it is important to balance increased load with rest and repair, and an efficient training plan schedules in recovery time. This chart illustrates the broad principles of applying training load.

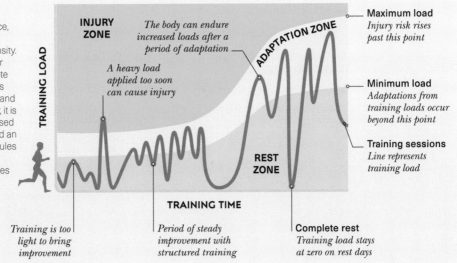

INJURY ZONE

The body can endure increased loads after a period of adaptation

A heavy load applied too soon can cause injury

ADAPTATION ZONE

TRAINING LOAD

REST ZONE

TRAINING TIME

Maximum load
Injury risk rises past this point

Minimum load
Adaptations from training loads occur beyond this point

Training sessions
Line represents training load

Training is too light to bring improvement

Period of steady improvement with structured training

Complete rest
Training load stays at zero on rest days

COMPETE

If you want to race and improve your times, you will have a much better chance of success if you follow a structured program to target a specific race. Targeted workouts can help develop your speed and teach you to pace yourself, while planning your training in phases will prepare you to perform at your peak on the day.

 ## STAY MOTIVATED

It can be difficult to stay motivated to run without a reason to keep striving. Following a training program provides you with a purpose for every workout, whether easy or hard. You have a reason to run at a specific pace, to run a specific distance, and to enjoy your easy runs as well. Many of us fall into a rut or reach a plateau if we do not have a way to monitor our progress; a training program helps you notice improvement, which is motivating in itself.

 ## ADD VARIETY

A good training plan will include workouts that vary in pace and distance, so there are fast, slow, short, and long runs. When you engage in varied, purposeful training and progressively higher training loads over time, your running form, speed, and fitness improves while keeping training varied and engaging.

YOUR **TRAINING GOALS**

Before you begin a training program, first consider what you want to achieve through training. Whether you are a complete beginner who is eager to train for your first race or an experienced runner who wants to take their training to the next level, it is useful to define some goals.

NEW TO RUNNING

If you are new to running or returning to it, setting a goal time or distance will give you something to work toward and measure your progress against. To achieve your goal, you will also need to attain a minimum level of fitness.

ACHIEVABLE GOALS

It is important to keep your first goals realistic—for example, running continuously for 3 miles

or for 30 minutes. If your eventual goals are ambitious, such as completing your first marathon, break them down into a series of targets or into A, B, and C goals to organize your priorities.

DEVELOPING FITNESS

Even if your ultimate goal is to run a marathon, your first objective should be to build up to a minimum base of aerobic and anaerobic

fitness (see below). Before starting a structured training program for the first time, you should be capable of doing short, hard sprints and easy continuous running over longer distances. When you can do both of these workout types, you can progress toward race-specific training. If you have not run before, the Beginner 5 km walk-run program (see pp.190–191) is a good place to start.

BUILDING A BASE
Before progressing to workout types that are more race-specific, establish a base level of aerobic and anaerobic fitness with easy continuous running (see p.180) and sprints (see p.188). The examples here show the workouts you should be able to complete before starting the Beginner 10 km program (see pp.192–193).

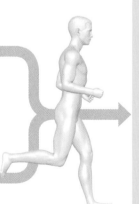

Aerobic base

Practice continuous running until you can complete these three workouts per week:

● Two 2-mile runs
● One 3-mile run

Anaerobic base

Practice strides (see p.87) until you can comfortably perform this workout 2–3 times per week:

● Four repetitions of **30-second strides** alternated by **1 minute walk**

Race-specific training

After you have established a base of fitness, you can start using a structured training program, which will include workouts such as:

● Longer easy continuous runs (see p.180)
● Fast continuous runs (see pp.181–183)
● Interval training (see pp.184–185)
● Hill training (see p.186)

FOUNDATION FITNESS

TRAINING FORM

TRAINING **FOR A RACE**

Once you have chosen a goal race distance, set a realistic time frame for reaching it, taking your current level of fitness into account.

INCREASING LOAD

When training for a race, your goals are to build volume by increasing the overall distance you run and to improve speed by increasing the intensity of your workouts.

Aim to increase your training load by 10–15 percent per week. The exact amount will depend on factors such as your training history and resilience, so it is important to keep monitoring your training load (see pp.168–169). Your highest loads should be undertaken 3–4 weeks prior to race day or 2–3 weeks prior for shorter races. After this point, you should "taper," or decrease training enough to ensure your body is fresh and ready to perform on race day.

PLANNING FOR RECOVERY

Following a race, give your body a period of active recovery by doing low-impact cross-training (see p.187) before preparing for another race. If you intend to run several races throughout the year, design a seasonal plan so that you peak for the important races and do not overreach. For complete recovery, it is also vital to have down periods during the year, or times when you focus on different types of running or alternative activities altogether.

ADVANCING YOUR TRAINING

You can advance your training by increasing the distance or the intensity of your workouts, or both.

As you progress, you will find that you can do the same training but with less effort, which is a sign of improved running economy (see p.165) and should result in improved race performance. Keep track of your training (see pp.168–169) and adjust your targets as you see improvements or if your workouts feel less challenging.

KEEPING UP MOMENTUM

Training usually follows a steplike progression. Increasing your training load will take effort at first, but as you become accustomed to it, your body will make physical adaptations (see p.159). Maintain your training level at a plateau until your body has absorbed the training load, then increase it once again.

ADDRESSING WEAKNESSES

Make sure to include all workout types (see pp.180–186) in your training plan. We tend to avoid workouts that address our weaknesses and are drawn to those that reveal our strengths. This becomes a self-fulfilling prophecy. It is a good idea to work on your weaknesses early in a training plan so that you are not scrambling to address a limitation in the weeks before a race.

TRAINING VOLUME

This graph shows the training volume per week in the Advanced Marathon training program (see pp.206–209). As this example shows, there should be periods of building and periods of recovery in every training plan.

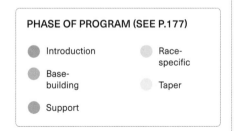

PHASE OF PROGRAM (SEE P.177)

- Introduction
- Base-building
- Support
- Race-specific
- Taper

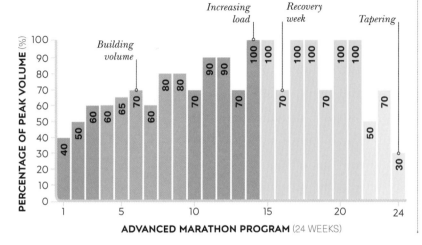

Building volume

Increasing load

Recovery week

Tapering

PERCENTAGE OF PEAK VOLUME (%)

40 50 60 60 65 60 80 80 70 90 90 70 100 100 70 100 100 70 100 100 50 70 30

ADVANCED MARATHON PROGRAM (24 WEEKS)

ASSESSING YOUR
FITNESS

It is important to assess your fitness at the beginning of a training regimen and then monitor its improvement as you continue. Fitness is measured by the level of intensity at which you can exercise and determines the appropriate level of workout for you. There are several methods you can use to measure intensity.

Health check

Get a health check-up if you are new to running or returning to it, especially if you have high blood pressure, diabetes, or heart or kidney disease. Also consult your physician if you have symptoms such as pain in the neck, chest, jaw, or arms; shortness of breath; dizziness or faintness; ankle swelling; or pain not relieved by rest.

MONITORING **EXERTION**

While high-tech equipment can measure intensity, simply rating exertion based on how you feel is proven to be highly effective.

The subjective effort you perceive as you exercise is directly related to how hard your heart and aerobic respiratory system are working. The fitter you are, the more intensely you can exercise at a low rate of perceived exertion (RPE). You should plan and monitor intensity on every run to ensure you train at the correct level and allow for adequate recovery.

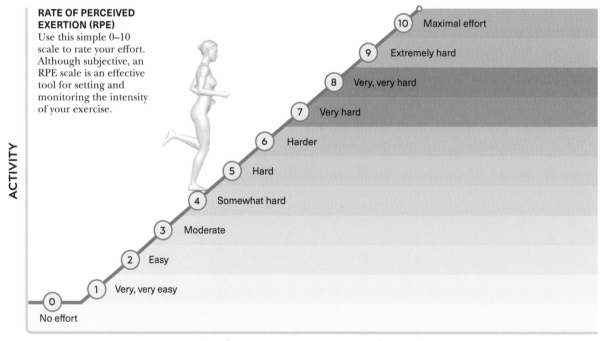

RATE OF PERCEIVED EXERTION (RPE)
Use this simple 0–10 scale to rate your effort. Although subjective, an RPE scale is an effective tool for setting and monitoring the intensity of your exercise.

ACTIVITY

10 Maximal effort
9 Extremely hard
8 Very, very hard
7 Very hard
6 Harder
5 Hard
4 Somewhat hard
3 Moderate
2 Easy
1 Very, very easy
0 No effort

RPE (RATE OF PERCEIVED EXERTION) SCALE

MONITORING **YOUR HEART RATE**

Heart rate elevates in a linear relationship with increasing effort, making it a good measure of exercise intensity.

Heart rate can indicate fitness if you track it over time. For example, if your pace at a given heart rate increases, it indicates that the pace is no longer as stressful as it once was. However, heart rate can be affected by fatigue, heat, terrain, and other variables, so use RPE alongside it during workouts.

HEART RATE IN TRAINING
During workouts, you can use a wrist or chest strap heart rate monitor to measure "heart rate reserve" (HRR). This is the range available to you for exercise and is the difference between your resting heart rate (RHR) and your maximum heart rate (see right). A higher resting heart rate can alert you to overtraining. The chart below shows the benefits of running at different percentages of heart rate reserve. Use the chart and formula below to calculate a target heart rate for a workout. For example, if your heart rate reserve is 110, your resting heart rate is 70, and your desired workout intensity is 85 percent of your heart rate reserve, (110 x 0.85) + 70 gives you a target heart rate of 163.5.

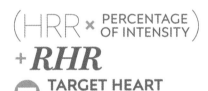

$$\left(HRR \times \frac{\text{PERCENTAGE}}{\text{OF INTENSITY}} \right)$$

$$+ \textbf{\textit{RHR}}$$

$$= \text{TARGET HEART RATE}$$

 Heart rate calculations
The heart is a muscle that becomes stronger with training. The lower your resting heart rate, the more efficient your heart is and the fitter you are. Maximum heart rate can help you monitor exertion.

CALCULATING YOUR RESTING HEART RATE
Before you get out of bed in the morning, take your pulse. Record this for several days to get a reliable average reading.

RESTING BEATS IN 10 SECONDS $\times$ **6**

$=$ **RESTING HEART RATE** (RHR)

CALCULATING YOUR MAXIMUM HEART RATE
The formula below provides an easy way to calculate your maximum heart rate. However, to account for your genetics and fitness level, a treadmill test (see p.167) is more accurate.

220 $-$ YOUR AGE

$=$ **MAXIMUM HEART RATE** (MHR)

CALCULATING YOUR HEART RATE RESERVE
To find out your heart rate reserve, use the simple calculation below. Your heart rate reserve may increase as your fitness improves.

MHR $-$ RHR

$=$ **HEART RATE RESERVE** (HRR)

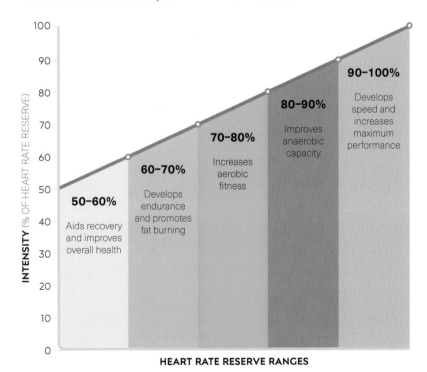

HEART RATE RESERVE RANGES

- **50–60%** Aids recovery and improves overall health
- **60–70%** Develops endurance and promotes fat burning
- **70–80%** Increases aerobic fitness
- **80–90%** Improves anaerobic capacity
- **90–100%** Develops speed and increases maximum performance

INTENSITY (% OF HEART RATE RESERVE)

Running power

You can buy wearable technology that estimates "running power" as a metric of intensity, but these have limitations. "Power" is used in cycling to calculate effort by measuring the mechanical power output of the legs. However, unlike in cycling, the relationship between mechanical power and metabolic energy consumption changes with conditions in running. For example, as you run uphill, the contribution of elastic energy from tendons decreases; on downhill runs, your muscles do less push-off and perform a braking action as you descend. Running-power meters are not able to measure these changes reliably, because they use estimates instead of true power readings.

MONITORING **PACE**

The pace of your workout is another measure of intensity, since increasing your speed involves increasing your effort.

A training program prescribes workouts at different goal paces to improve body systems such as aerobic efficiency and lactate clearance. A goal pace is the estimated speed in minutes per km or mile you must run to achieve a goal race time. Paces for longer distances are relatively slower than for short ones, because you must sustain them for longer. Doing workouts at different paces reveals your strengths and weaknesses. For example, if you can achieve a 5-km-pace workout but struggle with a half marathon–pace workout, this suggests you need to improve your endurance.

CALCULATING PACES

Online calculators can help you work out your goal paces over a range of distances (and are fairly accurate). They work by extrapolating from a recent race time or goal time you are training to achieve or your average time over a certain distance. During a workout, using a GPS device is the easiest way to measure your pace, but you can also feel your pace through effort (see opposite).

The chart below shows paces based on sample marathon goal times for different runners.

Pace calculator

	BEGINNER	IMPROVING RUNNER	ADVANCED RUNNER	ELITE RUNNER
MARATHON GOAL TIME	04:30:00	03:45:00	03:00:00	*WORLD RECORD* 02:01:39
Marathon pace	10:18/mile	8:35/mile	6:52/mile	4:39/mile
Half marathon pace	9:48/mile	8:10/mile	6:32/mile	4:25/mile
Lactate threshold pace	9:17/mile	7:52/mile	6:24/mile	4:25/mile
10-km pace	9:16/mile	7:43/mile	6:10/mile	4:10/mile
5-km pace	8:55/mile	7:26/mile	5:57/mile	4:01/mile
3-km pace	8:27/mile	7:03/mile	5:38/mile	3:48/mile
1500-m pace	7:55/mile	6:35/mile	5:16/mile	3:34/mile
800-m pace	7:12/mile	6:00/mile	4:48/mile	3:14/mile

COMPARING **RPE, HEART RATE, AND PACE**

Because they all measure effort, you can compare rate of perceived exertion (RPE), heart rate, and pace to assess your day-to-day and long-term fitness.

The relationship between RPE, heart rate, and pace is relative, since one runner's pace at RPE 4 will be different from another's. By keeping a record of your RPE, average heart rate, and average pace for each workout, you can learn what effort corresponds to a specific pace—for example, what 6:30 min/mile or your 10-km pace feels like and what heart rate range these paces fall into. However,

expect regular fluctuations in pace; if you are ill, fatigued, or stressed, your workout will feel harder.

Fitness will improve your pace at a particular heart rate or RPE score, or the pace will feel easier and result in a lower heart rate. If a pace feels harder and your heart rate increases, this can be a sign of fatigue or overtraining.

RPE AND PACE

The table shows approximate RPE scores for a range of paces. Because elite runners can run half marathon and 10 km paces harder and faster than recreational runners, this is reflected in the equivalent RPE.

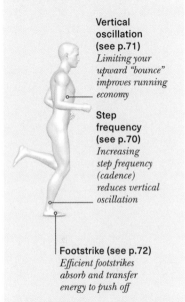

Running economy

The more economically a runner moves, the less oxygen they use at a given speed. A number of variables affect running economy, including genetics, environmental conditions, weight of clothing and shoes, fitness levels, and biomechanics. You can modify these last two factors through training, which is why improving your fitness and your running form (see pp.74–75) helps you run more efficiently at your goal pace.

Vertical oscillation (see p.71)
Limiting your upward "bounce" improves running economy

Step frequency (see p.70)
Increasing step frequency (cadence) reduces vertical oscillation

Footstrike (see p.72)
Efficient footstrikes absorb and transfer energy to push off

BIOMECHANICAL VARIABLES

RPE–pace equivalents

RPE	DESCRIPTOR	PACE/EFFORT
0	No effort	Sedentary
1	Very, very easy	Walking
2	Easy	Easy pace
3	Moderate	Marathon pace/half marathon pace (recreational)
4	Somewhat hard	Half marathon pace (elite)/lactate threshold pace/10-km pace (recreational)
5	Hard	10-km pace (elite)
6	Harder	5-km pace
7	Very hard	3-km pace
8	Very, very hard	1500-m pace
9	Extremely hard	800-m pace
10	Maximal effort	Sprinting/final exertion at the end of a race

FITNESS TESTS

Conducting fitness tests allows you to establish goals at the beginning of your training program and monitor improvements. To track your progress, you can repeat these tests, but the best way to measure your gains is to compete in a race. Lactate threshold (see pp.34–35) and VO₂ max (see p.37) are both good measures of fitness, which you can establish using one of the following field tests.

Calculating a benchmark LT pace

Although actual lactate threshold can vary from day to day, it is useful to use a benchmark LT pace for workouts where you need to run relative to LT pace—for example, 25 sec/mile slower than LT pace. You can generate an estimated LT pace by entering a recent race result into an online pace calculator (see p.164) or perform the following 30-minute time trial.

After a proper warm-up, gradually increase your pace to a level that is the fastest you can maintain for the full 30 minutes, then start the stopwatch. Measure your pace with a GPS device, or run on a treadmill or a measured track and calculate how far you run during the 30 minutes. Your current LT pace is 30 minutes divided by your total distance run. For example, if you run 5 miles in 30 minutes, your average LT pace is 6:00 min/mile.

Determining lactate threshold pace

Your lactate threshold (LT) pace is the highest possible speed you can run without causing an accumulation of blood lactate in your muscles. Training at LT pace raises this threshold, and your body adapts to perform aerobic cell respiration— which clears lactate—at faster paces.

Lactate threshold pace should stay just within the aerobic range of activity, which should feel like a "comfortably hard" pace that you could sustain for around 1 hour in race conditions. (LT pace is also called 1-hour race pace.) In order to train at your LT pace, you need to be able to recognize and monitor it so you can track improvements over time. Lactate threshold can be measured in a laboratory, but another simple way is to use the RPE scale (see p.162).

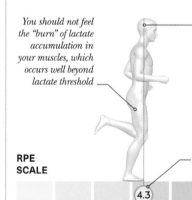

You should not feel the "burn" of lactate accumulation in your muscles, which occurs well beyond lactate threshold

Your lactate threshold pace
LT pace is an effort level and, as such, it will vary depending on the terrain, weather, altitude, and how you feel on the day

RPE 4.3
Running at your lactate threshold should feel comfortably hard; LT pace has been shown to correspond to RPE 4.3

RPE SCALE

4.3

Aerobic activity
Below LT pace, aerobic cell respiration allows your body to clear lactate faster than it accumulates

Anaerobic activity
Above LT pace, anaerobic cell respiration builds lactate faster than your body can clear it, causing hard breathing

RPE AND LACTATE THRESHOLD
Learn to feel when you are running at LT pace. It is a specific effort level reached by running as fast as you can without having to breathe hard. If you are breathing too hard, slow down.

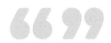

*The 0–10 RPE scale has a **direct** and **reliable** relationship with the lactate threshold and can be used to judge LT pace **on any run***

VO₂ max: treadmill test

This method to test VO₂ max requires you to run on a treadmill at a constant speed while the slope increases at 1-minute intervals, until you can no longer keep the pace. You will be pushing your body to its limits, so have an assistant adjust the treadmill slope for you. Use the total time you run to calculate your VO₂ max.

VO₂ max: Cooper test

This test, developed by Dr. Ken Cooper in 1968, offers a simple way to measure aerobic fitness. To complete it, simply run as far as you can in 12 minutes and use the total distance you have run to calculate your VO₂ max score using the formula below (using either the km or miles formula, as appropriate).

TIME MINUTES	SLOPE DEGREES
0	0°
1	2°
2	4°
3	6°
4	8°
5	10°
6	11°
7	12°
8	13°
9	14°
10	15°
11	16°
12	17°
13	18°
14	19°
15	20°

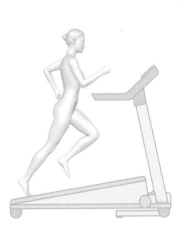

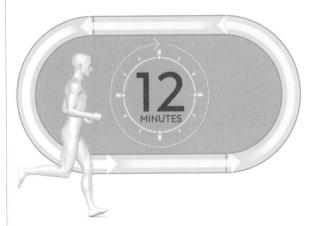

$$\left(42 + \text{TOTAL TIME RUN}\right) \times 2$$

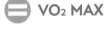 VO₂ MAX

$$\left(22.35 \times \text{TOTAL DISTANCE IN KM}\right) - 11.29$$

OR

$$\left(35.96 \times \text{TOTAL DISTANCE IN MILES}\right) - 11.29$$

VO₂ MAX

PERFORMING THE TEST

Set the treadmill to 7.02 mph (11.3 kph) and a slope of 0°. Every minute, the assistant increases the gradient according to the chart above. End the test when you cannot continue.

PERFORMING THE TEST

This test should be performed on a flat surface; a 440-yard (400-m) athletic track is ideal. Set your timer to count down from 12 minutes, run as far as possible, and record the total distance.

TRACKING
YOUR TRAINING

Most runners are good at tracking certain elements of their training either by keeping a log or recording their progress using a social media platform. Similarly, tools such as GPS watches, heart rate monitors, and other wearable devices can provide a wealth of information. There are various ways to benefit from this data.

WHY GATHER DATA?

Data can give you objective information about how your body is responding to training. If you collect the right data, it can both show areas of improvement and reveal which areas of training need more focus.

Collecting data is important for monitoring your health as well. It can provide information about how

your body is handling the training load and can alert you when you are at risk of overtraining or injury.

DATA TO RECORD

With the use of wearable devices (see box, opposite), you are able to gather a huge amount of data from your training. However, more is not always better—the key is to record the types of data that will help you

monitor your training load (see opposite), such as volume and intensity, and to observe your body's response to training through pain and fatigue scores. In addition, record which workout types (see pp.180–186) you do each week. Each has different benefits, so this will ensure you are including the right ingredients in your training.

Types of data

RPE, HEART RATE, AND PACE	**DISTANCE OR TIME**	**PAIN SCORE**	**FATIGUE SCORE**
Recording these factors (see pp.162–165) allows you to gauge the intensity, or effort level, of individual workouts. Over time, this data provides information about your fitness level, especially if you observe whether your heart rate or rate of perceived exertion (RPE) increases or decreases in relation to a given pace.	Monitoring these factors allows you to measure your volume. Not all miles are equal. Some runs are long and slow, while others are short and fast. A hill run may be shorter in distance than a flat run but take more time. In terms of gauging the physical toll of training, recording time is useful, but if training for a race, recording distance is also important.	Being attuned to any pain will allow you to pick up on patterns, which may help identify an injury early and aid in diagnosis and treatment. If you have any pain, record its location, its nature (using descriptors such as sharp, achy, tight), and its intensity. A simple scoring system of 0–10 will give you a very clear idea.	Fatigue is one of the first warning signs of overtraining syndrome. Rating how tired you feel after each workout (using a simple 0–10 scoring system) allows you to recognize rising fatigue levels and helps assess if you should include more recovery time in your training schedule.

MONITORING YOUR **TRAINING LOAD**

Training load refers to the total measure of stress applied to the body over time, which depends on the frequency, intensity, duration, and type of activity you do. Monitor your training load by giving each workout a score using the formula below. For example, if you perform hill runs at an effort rating of RPE 8 for 20 minutes, your training load score for the workout is 160. Record one internal and one external load (see below) consistently in order to aggregate the scores and track load over time.

Internal and external loads

Training load can be divided into two types: internal and external. External training load is an objective measure of volume, such as running 10 miles in distance or 60 minutes in duration. Internal training load represents the effort you put in to complete the workout, such as an average heart rate of 165 or an RPE of 4.

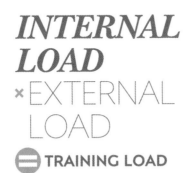

INTERNAL LOAD × EXTERNAL LOAD = **TRAINING LOAD**

Using tech to monitor progress

A wearable sensor such as a GPS-enabled wristwatch can be very convenient for collecting and logging multiple metrics. These devices can collect data about external training loads (such as distance, time, and elevation gain) and internal loads (such as heart rate and breathing rate). Some devices give real-time feedback, and many are paired with an online platform that can be used to track data longitudinally over time.

Other wearable devices can measure biomechanical variables such as cadence, impact, and vertical oscillation, which can be useful if you know how to interpret the data. However, be cautious about becoming too reliant on data at the cost of learning to run by feel.

Observing the changes

Two athletes may respond differently to the same training load, so it is important to regularly monitor yours. You can use pain and fatigue scores to observe whether your training load is improving your running or causing strain on your body. The body responds to the stress of the training load either by getting stronger or by breaking down, so any increases in load must be appropriate. Doing too much too soon may cause injury, but doing too little will not bring improvements.

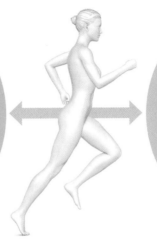

Signs of overtraining

Overtraining syndrome causes a sudden decline in performance, coordination, or strength, and fatigue that is not relieved by short rest. Signs include raised heart rate or RPE during workouts, elevated resting heart rate, appetite changes, weight loss, insomnia, irritability, lack of concentration, and depression. It is treated by reducing training load significantly or complete rest for weeks or months. Prevent it by spreading your training throughout the year and monitoring your overall training load.

Signs of improvement

The foremost sign of improvement, and often the most important for many runners, is faster race times. Additionally, if your average heart rate decreases at a given pace or if your RPE score becomes lower because the pace feels easier to you, it is a sign of improved fitness. Similarly, your pace at a given heart rate or RPE rating becomes faster as you become fitter. Other signs include a lower resting heart rate and the ability to manage higher weekly training loads.

TRAINING **TIPS**

At some point, either in your training or in a race, you will experience the urge to give up. Whether it is due to the pain in your legs, the doubt in your mind, or the overwhelming sense of fatigue, overcoming this sensation can be a defining moment for a runner and one that can make you stronger.

DEALING WITH PAIN

The pain of exertion is part of the running experience. It can take many forms: aching muscles deprived of glycogen, joints tested by repeated impacts, and running-related ailments ranging from blisters to stomach troubles.

In a race between two runners of seemingly equal physical talent, one runner's ability to overcome pain can give them an edge. Training is the best way to achieve this. Both trained and untrained runners have similar pain thresholds and will experience pain at the same point, but trained runners tend to have a higher pain tolerance and can withstand this pain for longer before easing off. How you feel pain doesn't alter, but training improves your ability to cope with it because your subconscious brain learns that your body can withstand the stress being placed on it (see below).

You can also affect pain consciously by using distraction techniques. Studies have shown that listening to fast-paced music while running can help you push your body further while your brain is occupied elsewhere.

The brain's response to exertion

These diagrams explore theories on how the brain decides the body can no longer bear the pain of exertion and whether the subconscious or conscious brain is the primary controller. Either way, training experience can modify the brain's response.

VOLUNTARY RESPONSE (CONSCIOUS BRAIN)
The conscious brain wants to stop activity due to perceived exertion or can spur the muscles to work harder in response to motivation stimulus.

MOTIVATION STIMULUS (EXTERNAL FACTOR)
Emotional motivation, such as a crowd cheering you on or the sight of the finish line, is registered by your conscious brain.

PERCEIVED EXERTION (CONSCIOUS BRAIN)
The conscious brain perceives fatigue, a perception generated by the subconscious brain after it has evaluated the pain signals.

CENTRAL GOVERNOR (SUBCONSCIOUS BRAIN)

MUSCLE CONTROL (PHYSICAL OUTCOME)
The subconscious brain regulates muscle recruitment to stop exercise before the body fails. However, the conscious brain also affects the decision to stop or continue.

PAIN STIMULUS (SUBCONSCIOUS BRAIN)
As you run, nerve signals travel from your muscles into the subconscious brain as pain stimuli, which are evaluated by the subconscious brain.

CENTRAL GOVERNOR MODEL
In this theory, a subconscious "governor" within the central nervous system generates the perception of fatigue and discomfort in order to halt the stress imposed on the body.

STAYING **MOTIVATED**

The motivation to train can come from a number of different sources. Learning to identify what motivates you to run, and to race, and reinforcing those motivations helps keep you on track to reach your goals.

A number of factors affect our motivation. In a race, the cheering of your family in the crowd or the anticipation of running a personal best can push you to dig a bit deeper into your energy reserves. In training, noticing the objective signs of improvement and completing challenging workouts in preparation for your race can motivate you to maintain your training load.

Visualizing yourself crossing the line and reaching your goal can help motivate you to train on a cold, wet day. One way to motivate yourself is to expect the pain and fatigue before it arrives and then embrace it when it does, knowing that pushing through it will only make you stronger for future workouts and races. Another more immediate and practical tool might be positive self-talk. Studies have shown that when things get tough, telling yourself, "You can do this" or "You can work through the pain" can improve your race performance.

Recognizing when you have dug deep enough and given your maximum effort is also important, so that you can give yourself adequate recovery time and avoid burnout (see right).

 Recovery and burnout

No athlete can sustain intense training indefinitely regardless of ability, experience, or mental toughness. You need to build recovery periods into your training schedule (see pp.174–175) or you risk burning out. The effects can include injury, poor training (leading to poor performance), low mood and sleep disorders, and illness. Proper recovery is important for allowing your body time to adapt to the training stimulus and get stronger, faster, and more efficient. However, recovery doesn't necessarily mean complete rest. Active recovery—such as light cycling, pool running, or swimming—is best, as it keeps your muscles and joints moving, but in a way that does not stress your body. That being said, sleep is the most powerful, evidence-based recovery tool.

MOTIVATION STIMULUS (EXTERNAL FACTOR)
Emotional motivation, such as a crowd cheering you on or the sight of the finish line, is registered by your conscious brain.

VOLUNTARY RESPONSE (CONSCIOUS BRAIN)
Your conscious brain spurs the muscles to work harder in response to motivation stimulus or wants to stop due to perceived fatigue.

MUSCLE CONTROL (PHYSICAL OUTCOME)
The conscious brain regulates muscle recruitment, making the decision of whether or not to terminate exercise.

PERCEIVED EXERTION (CONSCIOUS BRAIN)

PAIN STIMULUS (SUBCONSCIOUS BRAIN)
As you run, nerve signals travel from your muscles into the brain as pain stimuli, which are evaluated by the conscious brain.

PSYCHOLOGICAL-MOTIVATIONAL MODEL
This model proposes that the conscious brain decides when to stop running. This happens either when the effort required matches the maximal effort the runner is willing to exert or when the athlete believes they have exerted maximal effort and perceives that it is impossible to continue.

NUTRITION

Good nutrition is fundamental to your training. The primary nutrients to plan around are carbohydrates (essential for building up sufficient energy stores) and proteins (which help regenerate and repair muscle tissue after training).

Glycogen, which your body creates from carbohydrates, provides your primary fuel source during running. Your carbohydrate intake should therefore calibrate with your training load (see below).

It is best to maximize protein absorption and use by distributing your consumption of it through the day; aim to eat ½–¾ oz (15–20 g)

of protein 4–6 times a day. Lean animal protein is best, but plant sources (such as soy, legumes, and nuts) are also good.

POSTWORKOUT REFUELING

Following hard training sessions, it is important to eat foods that will help your body recover and refuel. Within 2 hours of a workout, aim to consume 1.5 g carbohydrate, 0.3 g protein, and 0.3 g fat per 2 pounds of your body weight. During the taper phase of training (see p.177), when energy expenditure is lower and you are trying to optimize body weight before a race, reduce the carbohydrate quantity to 1 g per 2 pounds of your body weight.

 ### Fueling before a run
Prerun meals should be high in carbohydrates to provide adequate fuel; pasta, rice, and other starches are ideal. After eating, you should allow 2–3 hours before working out to stop you from feeling bloated or getting a cramp. For runs longer than 90 minutes, or when muscle glycogen stores are low, you should take on approximately 1–2 oz (30–60 g) of carbohydrate per hour to maintain circulating glucose levels. This can be achieved through a combination of easily absorbed sports drinks; energy gels; or light, easily digestible, carbohydrate-rich foods such as energy bars. It is important to experiment with your nutrient sources—both the variety and intake levels—while you are still in training in order to find your optimal fuel intake for race day.

Changing nutrient needs

The harder you train, the more calories you will need to fuel your runs. Depending on the training phase (see p.177), your daily food intake should be 25–50 percent carbohydrates (ideally whole grains) to enable your body to generate optimal energy stores.

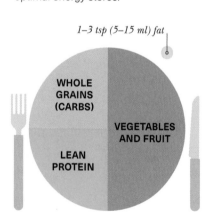

1–3 tsp (5–15 ml) fat

WHOLE GRAINS (CARBS)
VEGETABLES AND FRUIT
LEAN PROTEIN

Fruit
1–2 tbsp (15–30 ml) fat

WHOLE GRAINS (CARBS)
VEGETABLES
LEAN PROTEIN

Fruit
2–3 tbsp (30–45 ml) fat

GRAINS (CARBS)
LEAN PROTEIN **VEGETABLES**

EASY TRAINING
For light training—for example, in an introduction or taper phase—your total daily intake of carbohydrates need only be 25 percent, with fruits and vegetables making up the difference.

MODERATE TRAINING
As training increases—for example in the base-building or support phases of training—increase carbohydrate and fat intake. Additionally, fruit is recommended as a good source of carbohydrates.

HARD TRAINING OR RACE DAY
In a hard-training phase—such as the race-specific phase—carbohydrates should make up half of your daily food intake to allow your muscles to store more glycogen. This is known as "carb loading."

HYDRATION

There is no doubt that hydration is important when it comes to endurance running. It regulates body temperature through sweating, is essential to the transport of nutrients, and aids in releasing energy and removing waste products that are created by energy conversion.

Traditional wisdom had it that you should drink as much as possible prior to exercise. We now know that you do not need to drink copious amounts of water before a workout in order to stave off dehydration. Also untrue is the old belief that thirst signals indicate that you are already dehydrated. While drinking to thirst may not replace all the fluid lost during exercise (it is normal to lose up to 2–3 percent of your body weight during training sessions, or more during races), it is safer than the danger of overhydration (see box, right).

HYDRATION STRATEGIES

During a workout, responding to internal signals to drink when you are thirsty should be sufficient to keep you hydrated. If you sweat heavily during a run, or if it is a hot day, you may need to take in more fluids before a workout, but this should be weighed against the discomfort of having too much fluid in your stomach while running.

Sodium levels

Overhydration can be as dangerous as dehydration. During exercise, we lose sodium through sweating (known as electrolyte depletion). Drinking excessively during exercise dilutes the already depleted sodium levels in your blood. This can lead to sleep disruption and the potentially life-threatening condition Exercise Associated Hyponatremia (EAH). Symptoms include headaches, fatigue, nausea or vomiting, muscle spasms, and seizures.

Sports drinks contain electrolytes and therefore don't deplete the sodium levels in your blood in the same way that drinking water does. However, even drinking sports drinks to excess can dilute sodium levels.

Dehydration

Sweating during exercise will cause a certain amount of water loss from the body. If too much water is lost, however, it can affect your core temperature and energy supply to the muscles.

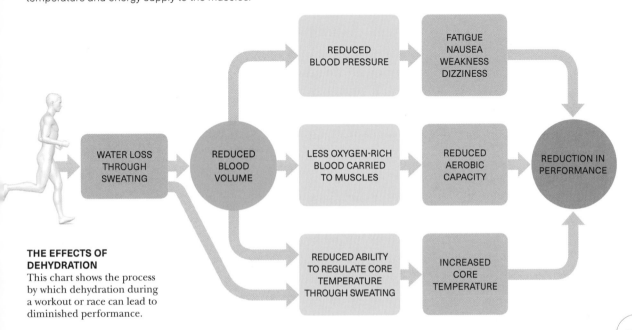

THE EFFECTS OF DEHYDRATION
This chart shows the process by which dehydration during a workout or race can lead to diminished performance.

RECOVERY AND REGENERATION

Scheduling recovery time is a vital part of training. It allows your body to renew energy reserves and cements the physiological adaptations that your body makes in response to training load.

"Active" recovery with low-impact, low-intensity activities between your main workouts keeps your muscles and joints mobile (see below). Massage, practicing mental resilience, and ensuring good sleep quality are other key ways to help the body recover.

A few other tools and therapies have shown positive effects on perceived postexercise muscle soreness: compression garments; cold water immersion (immersing legs in icy water for 10–15 minutes postexercise); contrast baths (immersing the legs alternately in tubs of warm and cold water for 20–30 minutes); and cryotherapy (applying cold, such as an ice pack, to muscles). Hyperbaric therapy, electrostimulation, and other trends, however, have little evidence to support their usefulness.

*Proper recovery is as important as, if not even **more important** than, training itself*

Mobility

After a hard training session, it can be tempting to stay fairly sedentary until your next workout. However, keeping your body mobile while still allowing it to recover—known as active recovery—can provide benefits, including an increase in your body's ability to clear metabolites such as blood lactate, improved muscle function, and reduced postexercise soreness. On days that are not scheduled for your key workouts (see p.179), keep your recovery time active with cross-training (see p.187); "recovery" runs at an easy pace (see p.180); or an exercise routine to keep your joints, muscles, and tendons moving (see right). All of these activities should be low in impact and intensity compared to your key workouts.

MOBILITY ROUTINE
You can build exercises into your daily routine at different times of day to keep your body mobile.

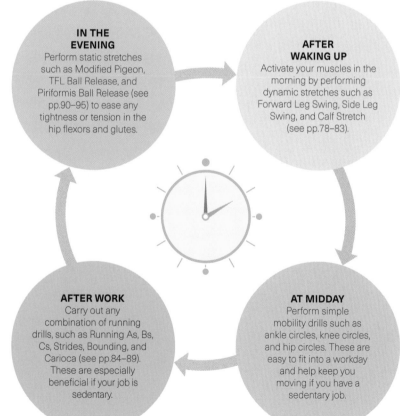

IN THE EVENING
Perform static stretches such as Modified Pigeon, TFL Ball Release, and Piriformis Ball Release (see pp.90–95) to ease any tightness or tension in the hip flexors and glutes.

AFTER WAKING UP
Activate your muscles in the morning by performing dynamic stretches such as Forward Leg Swing, Side Leg Swing, and Calf Stretch (see pp.78–83).

AFTER WORK
Carry out any combination of running drills, such as Running As, Bs, Cs, Strides, Bounding, and Carioca (see pp.84–89). These are especially beneficial if your job is sedentary.

AT MIDDAY
Perform simple mobility drills such as ankle circles, knee circles, and hip circles. These are easy to fit into a workday and help keep you moving if you have a sedentary job.

Massage

As your training load increases, you are likely to feel muscle tightness and stiffness in a number of areas of your body. One way to deal with this is to schedule regular massage therapy during your training.

Massage may help relax muscle tissue and reduce postexercise soreness. Although evidence suggests that it does not increase blood flow or help with removal of metabolic waste products (both often said to be benefits of massage), the positive psychological effects of massage are consistently reported in scientific studies. These include improvements in perceived recovery and perceived muscle soreness.

Massage also has an effect on the nervous system by helping activate the parasympathetic nervous system (see p.42), which is responsible for subduing the stress responses generated by working out and racing.

If you are unable to see a massage therapist regularly, consider self-massage. There are a number of tools available, such as foam rollers and lacrosse-style therapy balls, which can be used to target specific areas where you feel muscle tension. See also the TFL and Piriformis Ball Release stretches on pages 92–95.

Meditation

Practicing meditation can primarily benefit runners by aiding relaxation and stress relief. This in turn helps ensure restful sleep so your body can repair efficiently.

In addition, meditation encourages you to practice mental focus, which can boost willpower and self-discipline when you must motivate yourself to keep up your training regimen. It may also help increase your mental resilience when battling frustration, pain, stress, and tough training days and bolster you during racing challenges.

Sleep

The quality and quantity of sleep is the most important recovery factor for any runner. In fact, sleep deprivation can impact the performance of distance runners more than some other athletes. Suboptimal sleep affects the immune and endocrine systems—impacting recovery and training adaptation—and can also result in impaired cognitive function, increased pain perception, changes in mood, and altered metabolism. Endurance training has been shown to suppress immunity, so good sleep hygiene (see right) is vital to allow the immune system to recover. If sleep is cut short, the body does not have time to repair and consolidate memory. This can result in increased injury risk due to slower reaction times.

Sleep hygiene

Proper sleep hygiene can enhance sleep quality and quantity. Try the following habits and practices:

- Keep the bedroom dark, quiet, and cool at 66–70°F (19–21°C)
- Ensure your bed and pillow are comfortable
- Avoid backlit screens in the hour before bedtime
- Avoid caffeine later in the day
- Go to bed and wake up at the same time every day
- Create a nightly routine that starts 30 minutes before bedtime to prepare your body for sleep
- Use relaxation or breathing techniques (see Meditation, above) if you are anxious or have difficulty falling asleep

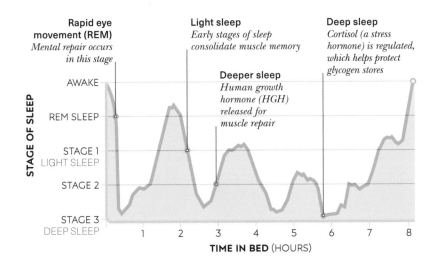

Rapid eye movement (REM)
Mental repair occurs in this stage

Light sleep
Early stages of sleep consolidate muscle memory

Deep sleep
Cortisol (a stress hormone) is regulated, which helps protect glycogen stores

Deeper sleep
Human growth hormone (HGH) released for muscle repair

STAGE OF SLEEP

AWAKE
REM SLEEP
STAGE 1 LIGHT SLEEP
STAGE 2
STAGE 3 DEEP SLEEP

1 2 3 4 5 6 7 8
TIME IN BED (HOURS)

SLEEP FOR RECOVERY
There are distinct stages of sleep, and we pass through each one several times a night. Each is essential for recovery.

CHOOSING AND USING A TRAINING PLAN

What makes a training program effective is whether it is the right stimulus for a runner at their current level of fitness and training. There are both beginner and advanced training programs included in this book, designed to give you a structure of key workouts that you can build upon and adapt if you wish.

TYPES OF PROGRAMS

The training programs in this chapter include beginner programs for 5 km, 10 km, half marathon, and marathon, as well as advanced programs for 10 km, half marathon, and marathon.

BEGINNER PROGRAMS

If you have not run before, have not run for long time, or are returning to training after injury, you can start with the Beginner 5 km Program. This is designed in a walk-run format to gradually build up the length of time you can run continuously. Once you have graduated from completing your first 5 km run, you may choose to work toward longer distances.

There is no rule that you need to continue progressing in distance, however. Many runners prefer to stick to shorter distances and work on improving their finishing time. That said, if your body is able to absorb the training load for each successive distance level, it can be satisfying to continue. Over their 12-week time frames, the beginner programs primarily focus on your ability to complete the target distance.

ADVANCED PROGRAMS

The advanced programs are suitable for those who have already completed a race at the goal distance and are looking to improve their finishing time.

Compared to the beginner programs, the advanced training programs include more overall volume and intensity, as well as more variety and complexity of workouts. In order to build up to a higher level of fitness over the course of the programs, they progress over 24 weeks rather than just 12 weeks. This longer time period allows for an introduction phase (see opposite) within these programs, and there is time to focus on achieving particular goals in each phase, with shifts in the types of workouts being performed.

PROGRAM PROGRESSION
Each of the 12-week beginner programs (5 km, 10 km, half marathon, and marathon) progress from where the previous program finished. This means it is possible to follow these 4 programs all the way through from a starting point of no running to completing a marathon within 48 weeks.

BEGINNER 5 KM PROGRAM	BEGINNER 10 KM PROGRAM	BEGINNER HALF MARATHON PROGRAM	BEGINNER MARATHON PROGRAM
WEEKS 1–12 (see pp.190–191)	WEEKS 13–24 (see pp.192–193)	WEEKS 25–36 (see pp.198–199)	WEEKS 37–48 (see pp.204–205)

TRAINING **PHASES**

The training programs in this book are divided into phases. The phases gradually shift from a focus on developing general aerobic and anaerobic fitness toward workouts that are specific for your target event. The cycle here shows the typical number of weeks spent in each phase in a 24-week program.

INTRODUCTION PHASE

Start with an introduction phase if you have just completed a hard race or training period. (This phase appears in advanced programs only.) The aim of this phase is to refresh you physically and mentally before rebuilding your general running volume to a level that allows for more focused training to begin. The programs allocate 3 weeks to this phase, but it can be extended by weeks, months, or even a rest from running, depending on your level of fatigue.

TAPER

At the end of the race-specific phase is the taper before your race. You cannot perform at your best when your level of training fatigue is at its highest, even though your fitness may be at its peak. On the flip side, you cannot perform your best if your fitness has dropped too far. The art of the taper is therefore to perform workouts that allow you to arrive at the starting line as fresh as possible while simultaneously offering enough volume and intensity to maintain your fitness.

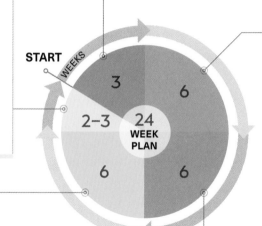

BASE-BUILDING PHASE

For both beginners and advanced runners, the focused training begins in this phase. The goal is to increase your aerobic volume; gradually introduce intensity; and improve running skills such as form, strength, power, cadence, and sprinting ability. This is the best phase to work on your own weaknesses, whether that is speed, strength, or endurance. Regardless of the end distance being targeted, the goal of this phase is to become a fitter, faster, and stronger overall runner.

RACE-SPECIFIC PHASE

This is the phase that focuses on the specific demands of your target race with peak workouts and long runs. Your capacity to run both fast and long should now be developed, and the emphasis is on making your goal race pace feel as efficient as possible. The workouts mainly target the dominant energy system that will be utilized during your target race. In the advanced programs, you will have reached peak volume (see p.188) in the support phase and adapted to it, leaving you with more energy to put into the workouts.

SUPPORT PHASE

The main goal of this phase is to prepare you for the race-specific phase to come. The support phase builds upon the general fitness established in the previous phase and begins to focus on workouts that support the race distance and pace that you are training toward. There are workouts faster than your goal race pace designed to make your actual goal race pace feel more comfortable by comparison. There are also slower workouts that help build your endurance and your ability to sustain your goal race pace over the target distance.

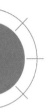

TRAINING
PRINCIPLES

These principles should inform the structure of a successful training plan. They are proven effective for all runners, from recreational to elite, and understanding them will help you get the most from your training program and workouts.

Well-rounded fitness

Focus on improving overall general fitness with anaerobic and form-training workouts, as well as aerobic running fitness, to become a more well-rounded runner.

Progressive adaptation

Gradually introduce different training stimuli to promote physical adaptations by changing the volume, intensity, or frequency of workouts.

Increase intensity

Make workouts harder in one of four ways: increasing the pace, increasing the distance or duration of a run at a given pace, increasing the ratio of fast to slower running, or running recovery sections faster.

Increase volume

Progressively increase the volume of running to a predetermined peak over the course of a training program, with some weeks decreasing in volume to allow your body to absorb the training load.

Optimize training load

Your training load should increase at a rate that your body can absorb and benefit from. Monitor for signs of overtraining (see pp.168–169) and adjust if needed.

WORKOUT TYPES

Performing a variety of workout types will help make you a well-rounded runner, as well as help you become stronger and fitter.

The workouts in the programs range from short sprints to longer aerobic-based running. Four main categories of workout are described: easy continuous running, fast continuous running, interval training, and hill training (see pp.180–186). This is one system of categorizing workouts—you may come across others. Each of these workout types provides different benefits in terms of increasing endurance, speed, and strength.

In addition, there are form-focused interval workouts that help improve your running form (see p.188).

INDIVIDUALIZATION

Due to the range of types, you may find some workouts more difficult than others. If a pattern emerges, you may identify that you are an endurance-based runner rather than a speed-based runner, or vice versa. The training programs should not be seen as set in stone. This means that if you identify a weakness early in your training cycle, you can shift the emphasis of your training by choosing workout types that address your weakness.

Depletion training

This type of training involves running in a glycogen-depleted state in order to improve the body's ability to metabolize fat. This is useful for race events that last longer than 90 minutes (the average length of time that muscle glycogen can provide you with fuel when running).

The easiest way to achieve this glycogen-depleted state is to schedule your run before breakfast (ensuring at least 10 hours of fasting overnight). After a depletion run, it is important to replenish muscles with a high-carbohydrate recovery meal.

Depletion training is stressful and should be undertaken with caution. Introduce it early in the training cycle and begin with just one session per week; you can add more as your body adapts. Reduce or omit these runs completely in the taper period.

PLANNING YOUR TRAINING

The programs in this book show three key workouts per week: two shorter, more intense workouts and one longer run.

These key workouts should be the most stressful training stimuli of your week. Only three are scheduled per week to allow at least one recovery day between each key workout. Depending on your level of experience, fitness, and available time, a recovery day could involve full rest, cross-training (see p.187), or easy continuous running (see p.180). However, keep in mind that any recovery day activity should be easy enough that you feel ready to run the distance and effort prescribed in your next key workout.

Performing the three key workouts each week will serve you well, but if you want to train more often than 3 days a week and add to the key workouts in your schedule, bear in mind that it is easier to recover from multiple short runs than from a smaller number of long runs. Compared to the longest run of the week, your second-longest run should be no more than half its distance or duration, and any remaining runs should not be more than one-third.

KEY

··········	Short run
‖‖‖‖	Medium run
‖‖‖‖‖	Long run
·//////‖	Progression run
‖-‖-‖-‖-	Pace-change run
·‖·‖·‖·	Anaerobic capacity training
⌐⌐⌐	Hill run

STRUCTURING YOUR WEEK
The examples below show how to fit extra sessions in between key workouts, if you choose. It is best to stick to easy continuous runs and cross-training.

BEGINNER RUNNER

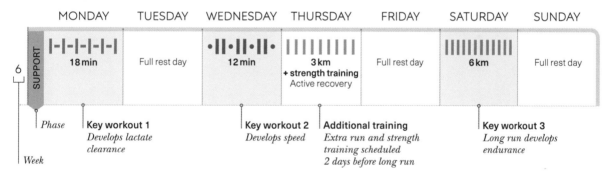

	MONDAY	TUESDAY	WEDNESDAY	THURSDAY	FRIDAY	SATURDAY	SUNDAY
SUPPORT (Week 6)	‖-‖-‖-‖- 18 min	Full rest day	·‖·‖·‖· 12 min	‖‖‖‖‖‖‖ 3 km + strength training Active recovery	Full rest day	‖‖‖‖‖‖‖‖ 6 km	Full rest day

Phase | **Key workout 1** *Develops lactate clearance* | | **Key workout 2** *Develops speed* | **Additional training** *Extra run and strength training scheduled 2 days before long run* | | **Key workout 3** *Long run develops endurance* |

ADVANCED RUNNER

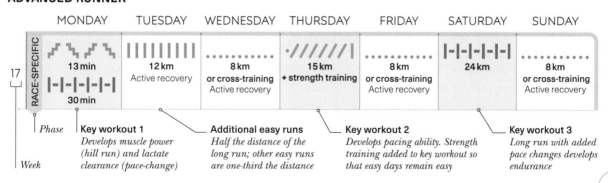

	MONDAY	TUESDAY	WEDNESDAY	THURSDAY	FRIDAY	SATURDAY	SUNDAY
RACE-SPECIFIC (Week 17)	⌐⌐⌐ 13 min ‖-‖-‖-‖- 30 min	‖‖‖‖‖‖‖‖ 12 km Active recovery	·········· 8 km or cross-training Active recovery	·//////‖ 15 km + strength training	·········· 8 km or cross-training Active recovery	‖-‖-‖-‖- 24 km	·········· 8 km or cross-training Active recovery

Phase | **Key workout 1** *Develops muscle power (hill run) and lactate clearance (pace-change)* | **Additional easy runs** *Half the distance of the long run; other easy runs are one-third the distance* | | **Key workout 2** *Develops pacing ability. Strength training added to key workout so that easy days remain easy* | | **Key workout 3** *Long run with added pace changes develops endurance* |

EASY CONTINUOUS
RUNNING

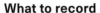

What to record

- Distance
- Duration
- Average pace
- RPE score

The subjective effort of these runs should be the focus more than the pace. Make sure they are "easy."

This type of training is performed at the lowest effort level of all workout types and makes up the bulk of training volume for distance runners. Depending on distance or duration, easy continuous runs are classified in this book as "short," "medium," or "long," which are definitions relative to your experience.

DISTANCE AND RECOVERY RUNS

The purpose of easy continuous running is to build a strong aerobic base without placing too much extra load on top of the more intense workouts in a training program.

BENEFITS

The cumulative volume of easy continuous running improves endurance; increases capillaries and mitochondria (see pp.34–35);

and, in the case of long runs, gives you confidence that you can complete the distance of the target event.

HOW TO DO IT

These runs are done at "easy pace," which means they should be run as slowly as needed to maintain good form and relaxation throughout the session. They should also help you achieve

adequate recovery before your next workout, so it is helpful to set a pace or effort limit (for example, no higher than 70 percent of heart rate reserve) to ensure they remain easy.

At the start of a program, the long run should build up to a set distance. Once this is achieved, you can increase the training load with pace variations (making them fast continuous runs) or increase the distance without intensity.

Types and frequency

These three types of easy continuous running workouts are described in terms of relative distance or duration. Bear in mind that as you progress, what was once a "long" run may become a medium run. How frequently you do these three types of easy continuous running will depend on your level of experience, training phase, and distance target. Some elite runners perform one easy continuous run a day.

SHORT RUNS

Compared to the longest run in your training plan, short runs are usually one-third the distance or duration (or less).

Short runs are typically scheduled in between more challenging efforts, either to begin or finish a workout, or on a recovery day for advanced runners (which is termed a "recovery run"). Short runs may also be a workout in their own right in a light training week.

MEDIUM RUNS

These runs are between one-third and half the distance or duration of the longest run in your training plan.

These runs can be done once a week in addition to the weekly long run. Follow with at least 1 day of rest or a recovery run (see short runs). This "extra" run is particularly useful for marathoners, as it helps increase aerobic volume, especially if you run only 3–4 times a week.

LONG RUNS

This is the longest run of the week. It can be defined as any run that is 50 percent of the distance or duration of the longest run in your training plan, or more.

Include one long run per week, particularly during the base-building phase. Later in the program, long runs can evolve into fast continuous runs by including pace variations, especially for half marathoners and marathoners.

FAST CONTINUOUS RUNNING

These runs are done faster than easy pace but not so fast or sustained that you need to stop or walk to recover. Therefore, there is an element of control involved in this type of training. The three basic types of fast continuous runs are tempo runs, progression runs, and pace-change runs.

/IIIIII\ TEMPO RUNS

Tempo runs are even-paced runs, typically run at speeds from lactate threshold pace at the faster end to a little under marathon pace at the slower end (see box). Tempo runs are sometimes preceded or followed by a short, easy run for warm-up or recovery.

BENEFITS

These workouts teach you how to run at a constant, sustainable pace or effort over a set distance or duration. Besides racing, no other workout develops an awareness of pace as efficiently

as a tempo run. They also increase aerobic capacity and the rate of lactate clearance.

HOW TO DO IT

Complete these runs at an even pace or effort for the whole run. The first tempo runs in your program may be slower than goal pace (the speed you are trying to achieve) so that you can start at a manageable effort level and pace. This is known as "date pace"—the pace you can sustain at the current date. As your fitness improves, the pace of the tempo run can progress to goal pace.

Example

The examples below show the typical distance or duration for tempo runs at the following efforts and paces.

LACTATE THRESHOLD

Run at or faster than your lactate threshold pace (see pp.166–167) for 20–40 minutes.

20–40 min @ **LT**

HALF MARATHON PACE

Run at half marathon goal pace for 5–10 miles.

5–10 miles @ **HMP**

MARATHON PACE

Run at marathon goal pace for 8–16 miles.

8–16 miles @ **MP**

Effort-based and distance-based paces

On average, lactate threshold (LT) pace correlates to the pace you can maintain for 1 hour in a competition. This is why LT pace is sometimes called 1-hour race pace. Because marathons and half marathons (for most runners except elite) take much longer than an hour to complete, marathon and half marathon paces are slower than LT pace, so that they can be sustained over a longer distance. Similarly, half marathon pace is usually faster than marathon pace, because it is a shorter event. Your training program will contain various distance-based paces (not just the goal pace for your target event) so that you run relatively slower or faster as appropriate for the workout. (See pp.164–167 for how to calculate paces for training purposes.)

·///////⟍ PROGRESSION RUNS

These runs increase in pace or effort incrementally over the course of the run. For example, a 30-minute run can increase in pace every 6 minutes.

BENEFITS

Progression runs teach you how to feel your pace and increase it, even when you are tired. Physiologically, these workouts increase the oxygen uptake in a higher percentage of muscle fibers, accelerating turnover by engaging first the slow-twitch muscles fibers, then the fast-twitch fibers (see p.19) in the later stages of the run.

HOW TO DO IT

These runs are typically performed at a slower average pace compared to an equivalent tempo run due to the demands of acceleration on the muscles and aerobic system. The duration or distance of a progression run tends to be split into 2–5 segments; these are assigned paces that increase by 5–15 sec/mile per segment. The overall average pace is as important as that of the individual segments, so the first progression runs in your program can be relatively easy overall and become faster as your fitness improves.

Examples

The examples below show the typical pace or effort for runs of the following durations and distances.

30-MINUTE PROGRESSION

Run 5 segments of 6 minutes each, averaging 8–16 sec/mile slower than your lactate threshold (LT) pace (see p.166).
    This example starts at 24 sec/mile slower than LT pace and ends at 8 sec/mile faster than LT pace.

·///////⟍
5 x 6-min runs
@ 24 sec < LT
+ @ 16 sec < LT
+ @ 8 sec < LT
+ @ LT
+ @ 8 sec > LT

10-MILE PROGRESSION

Run 5 segments of 2 miles each, averaging 15 sec/mile slower than your half marathon goal pace.
    This example starts at 45 sec/mile slower than half marathon pace and ends at 15 sec/mile faster than half marathon pace.

·///////⟍
5 x 2-mile runs
@ 45 sec < HMP
+ @ 30 sec < HMP
+ @ 15 sec < HMP
+ @ HMP
+ @ 15 sec > HMP

16-MILE PROGRESSION

Run 4 segments of 4 miles each, averaging 16 sec/mile slower than your marathon goal pace.
    This example starts at 40 sec/mile slower than marathon pace and ends at 8 sec/mile faster than marathon pace.

·///////⟍
4 x 4-mile runs
@ 40 sec < MP
+ @ 24 sec < MP
+ @ 8 sec < MP
+ @ 8 sec > MP

Frequency

Fast continuous runs can be performed up to three times per week, depending on your level of experience, training phase, and goal distance. During the base-building phase (see p.177), a short and a long easy continuous run can evolve into a tempo, progression, or pace-change run. In later phases, race preparation will determine the number of these progression runs needed per week.

5 KM GOAL DISTANCE

When your target distance is 5 km, a good guide is to include fast continuous runs up to twice a week during the base-building phase, once a week during the support phase, and once every 2 weeks during the race-specific phase.

10 KM GOAL DISTANCE

For this target distance, you will benefit from including tempo, progression, or pace-change runs up to twice a week. These fast continuous runs can be done throughout the base-building, support, and race-specific phases.

|-|-|-|-| PACE-CHANGE RUNS

As the name suggests, pace-change runs involve alternating between slower and faster paces during a continuous run. They can be done over any distance or duration, and the pace variations can be structured or spontaneous.

BENEFITS

These runs teach the body to run fast without complete recovery. If the fast sections are run faster than lactate threshold, causing lactate to build up, the slow-twitch muscles that are activated in the slower sections clear the lactate accumulation. This improves your muscles' ability to use lactate as fuel.

HOW TO DO IT

When you begin pace-change runs, there may be only 5–10 minutes of fast running within your continuous run. As your fitness improves, you can increase the volume or the pace of the fast sections, the volume of the overall run, or the pace of the slower "recovery" sections. Being able to keep the pace of the recoveries close to the fast pace or to decrease their duration indicates that your muscles have improved their ability to clear lactate.

Examples

The examples below show typical workouts from a range of training programs.

LACTATE THRESHOLD (LT) PACE

Run for 30 minutes, alternating 3 minutes at 15 sec/mile faster than LT with 2 minutes at 25 sec/mile slower than LT.

30 min
⋈ **3 min @ 15 sec >** LT **with**
2 min @ 25 sec < LT

HALF MARATHON-SPECIFIC

Run for 10 miles, alternating 2 miles at half marathon pace with 0.5 mile at 50 sec/mile slower than half marathon pace.

|-|-|-|-|
10 miles
⋈ **2 miles @** HMP **with**
0.5 mile @ 50 sec < HMP

FARTLEK

Meaning "speed play" in Swedish, fartlek runs are less structured than other pace-change runs, with the pace variations done spontaneously as you run.

A typical fartlek run might last for 45 minutes, alternating between hard, fast sections that last 15 seconds to 3 minutes and easy recovery sections. The recoveries should last 1–2 times the duration of the fast sections.

6-MILE GOAL-SPECIFIC

Run for 6 miles, alternating 1.5 miles at 10-km goal pace with 0.5 mile at 50 sec/mile slower than 10-km goal pace.

|-|-|-|-|
6 miles
⋈ **1.5 miles @** 10km **with**
0.5 mile @ 50 sec < 10km

MARATHON-SPECIFIC

Run for 15 miles, alternating 2.5 miles at marathon goal pace with 0.5 mile at 40 sec/mile slower than marathon goal pace.

|-|-|-|-|
15 miles
⋈ **2.5 miles @** MP **with**
0.5 mile @ 40 sec < MP

HALF MARATHON GOAL DISTANCE

When you are training for a half marathon, a good rule of thumb is to include fast continuous runs up to twice a week during the base-building and support phases. You can increase this to up to three times a week during the race-specific phase.

MARATHON GOAL DISTANCE

Do fast continuous runs up to twice a week during base-building and up to three times a week in later phases. To improve speed, reduce these workouts in the support phase and focus on VO2 max training (see p.184). If your 5 km and 10 km race times are fast, focus on fast continuous running to improve your running economy and ability to clear lactate.

INTERVAL
TRAINING

What to record

- RPE score for each repetition
- Average time or pace of each repetition
- Individual time or pace for each repetition (Note whether the paces were consistent or whether the pace increased or slowed down throughout the workout.)

The focus of interval training is the intensity of the fast sections, so keep track of the repetitions.

Also known as repetition training, interval training involves alternating periods of fast running with periods of recovery. The fast sections are intense, and the recoveries are light. It is performed at various intensity levels, but anaerobic capacity and VO₂ max are most important for distance runners.

 ## VO₂ MAX TRAINING

The intensity of these workouts is lower than anaerobic capacity interval training (see opposite) but higher than lactate threshold. Long fast sections alternate with relatively short recovery periods, which are of equal or half the duration of the fast sections.

BENEFITS

VO₂ max training improves the heart's ability to pump a higher volume of blood and the muscles' capacity to absorb more oxygen, thereby increasing your VO₂ max. It improves speed over 5-km and

10-km distances and helps marathoners who are slower over short distances and are plateauing at their marathon pace. Marathoners with fast 5-km and 10-km race times will be better served with training that is closer to lactate threshold.

HOW TO DO IT

The intensity of these workouts typically correlates with RPE 6–7, a heart rate reserve of 91–94 percent, or 3-km to 5-km race pace. The hard sections last between 20–2000 m (or 30 seconds to 6 minutes in duration).

Example

This shows repetitions for 3-km pace, but 5-km pace is also common.

3-KM PACE REPETITIONS

In this example, 4800 m is divided into 6 repetitions. Each recovery is equal in duration to each fast run (shown by 1 circle). If you average 2.5 minutes per run, each recovery would be 2.5 minutes of walking.

800 m @ 3km
+ ● walk
x6

Frequency

As a general rule, you should not begin sustained anaerobic capacity or VO₂ max workouts until the support phase (see p.177), after you have laid a foundation of strength and good running mechanics in the base-building phase. Doing longer hill repeats (see p.186) of 30 seconds to 4 minutes will help in this respect. How frequently you should include interval training in your regime depends on your goal distance.

5 KM GOAL DISTANCE

Anaerobic capacity Perform 10–30-second effort-based reps once a week during the base-building phase. During the support phase, do longer reps every second week.

VO₂ max During the support phase, perform 3-km pace reps every second week. As you prepare for your race in the race-specific phase, perform reps at 3-km pace or 5-km pace (or both) every week.

10 KM GOAL DISTANCE

Anaerobic capacity Perform 10–30-second effort-based reps once a week during the base-building phase. During the support phase, switch to 1500-m pace reps every second week.

VO₂ max During the support phase, perform reps at 3-km pace or 5-km pace every second week. As you prepare for your race in the 10-km race-specific phase, perform reps at 5-km pace every second week.

Intensity and recovery

Interval training and pace-change runs (see p.183) both alternate fast running with slower recoveries. However, interval training is focused on the intensity of the fast sections, while in pace-change runs, the pace of the recovery sections is equally important.

The rest periods in interval training are much slower than in pace-change runs, allowing your muscles to recover at a faster rate. This lets you do a high volume of fast, intense running within a shorter space of time, which improves the ability of your muscles to clear lactate. Interval training should be done on an even, level surface to allow you to maximize your pace as you train.

The two types of interval training recommended for distance runners—anaerobic capacity training and VO₂ max training—are both anaerobic workouts during which lactate builds up in the muscles (see pp.34–35). Therefore, the recovery intervals need to be slow enough to clear the lactate in preparation for the next high-intensity section.

•ll•ll•ll• ANAEROBIC CAPACITY TRAINING

This type of interval training is performed at a level of intensity that results in very high levels of lactate in the muscles. Short fast sections are interspersed with longer recovery periods lasting 2–4 times the duration of the fast sections.

BENEFITS

This workout helps increase the amount of energy produced by the anaerobic energy system. The high effort involved in anaerobic capacity training has a direct effect on improving speed over shorter distances, so it benefits 5-km and 10-km goal distances most. For half marathon and marathon training, hill reps at 100 percent intensity (see p.186) may be more beneficial.

HOW TO DO IT

Perform the fast sections at the fastest pace you can maintain without slowing down as the workout progresses. This will result in a heart rate value close to 100 percent by the end of the workout and an RPE of 8–9. (Only flat-out sprinting and the final burst in a race have a higher RPE score.)

Example

This shows intervals for 800-m pace, but 1500-m pace is also common.

800-M PACE REPETITIONS

In this example, 1600 m is divided into 4 repetitions. Each recovery is 4 times the duration of each fast run (shown by 4 circles). If you average 1 minute per run, each recovery would be 4 minutes of walking.

HALF MARATHON GOAL DISTANCE
Anaerobic capacity Perform short 10–30-second effort-based reps once a week during base-building. You do not need longer reps unless doing a 5-km or 10-km race in the same cycle. If so, discontinue them by the marathon race-specific phase.

VO₂ max In the support phase only, perform reps at 5-km pace every second week. Add in reps at 3-km pace if you are competing in a 5-km or 10-km race during the course of the training cycle.

MARATHON GOAL DISTANCE
Anaerobic capacity Perform 10–30-second reps once a week during base-building. Don't do longer reps unless you are racing 5 km or 10 km while marathon training, but end them by marathon race-specific phase.

VO₂ max To improve speed over 5 km and 10 km, perform reps at 3-km pace and 5-km pace every second week. Those racing 5 km or 10 km while marathon training, perform VO₂ max intervals in the support phase, but end them by marathon race-specific phase.

What to record

- Average pace of repetitions
- Heart rate for each uphill run
- RPE score for each uphill run
- Pace for each uphill run (Note whether they were consistent or if they increased or decreased throughout the session.)

As long as you use the same hill, monitoring pace helps track improvement. Record your heart rate and RPE to gauge effort.

HILL
TRAINING

You can perform hill training either by running up and down a gradient or over rolling terrain. It can be done at any effort and duration. You can perform intervals, fast continuous runs, and even long runs on hills. Unless you only race on the flat, hill training is a must to prepare you fully for your target event.

 HILL RUNS

The increased effort required by hill training improves aerobic and muscular conditioning, race preparation, and running form.

BENEFITS

Hill training engages a high percentage of muscle fibers, leading to increased muscular power. In particular, it strengthens muscles around the knee, as uphill running works the calves, hamstrings, and glutes, while downhill running puts more emphasis on the quadriceps. Hill training is a great way to improve the elements of good running form (see pp.74–75). Emphasizing tall posture, a slight forward lean, a high cadence, and striking the ground beneath your center of mass helps you overcome ground resistance running uphill while also

Examples

These examples show the typical duration of repetitions and recoveries for hill workouts of different intensities. Use these examples as a guide if you wish to convert a workout from level to hilly terrain.

UPHILL SPRINTS	DOWNHILL SPRINTS	HILLS AT ANAEROBIC CAPACITY	HILLS AT VO₂ MAX	HILLS AT LACTATE THRESHOLD
↑ 8–15-sec run @ 100 + ↓ 2-min walk — x4–10 —	↓ 15–30-sec run + ↑ 45 sec–2-min walk — 3–10 min —	↑ 15-sec–2-min run @ AC + ↓ 45-sec–6-min jog — 3–16 min —	↑ 30-sec–6-min run @ VO₂ + ↓ 1–12-min jog — 9–36 min —	↑ 1–8-min run @ LT + ↓ 1–12-min walk — 20–40 min —
Sprint uphill at 100 percent intensity (RPE 10) for 4–10 repetitions lasting 8–15 seconds each, with full recovery (typically 2 minutes or more walking) between each sprint. Ideal incline: 10–20%	This workout is good for improving running form. Perform 15–30-second runs downhill for a total of 3–10 minutes. Uphill recoveries should last 3–4 times the duration of the downhill run. Ideal incline: 3–8%	Perform 15-second to 2-minute runs uphill for a total of 3–16 minutes. Downhill recoveries should last 3 times the duration of the uphill run. Ideal incline: 5–10%	Perform 30-second to 6-minute runs uphill for a total of 9–36 minutes. Downhill recoveries should last twice the duration of the uphill run. Ideal incline: 5–10%	Perform 1–8-minute runs uphill for a total of 20–40 minutes. Downhill recoveries should ideally be of equal duration, which is very challenging but helps improve lactate clearance. Ideal incline: 3–6%

Frequency

For most runners, the extra intensity and workload of hill runs will mean replacing another key workout.

HILL RUNS

As hard workouts, hill runs should count among your three key weekly workouts (see p.179), so you would not generally perform them more than three times a week. However, if you do run between key training days, keep any extra hill runs very easy. If you are training for a hilly event, consider converting more of your workouts to hill training.

decreasing impact forces as you run downhill. Performing vigorous, short-hill sprints can also increase heart stroke volume (the amount of blood pumped by the heart in a single contraction).

HOW TO DO IT

Find a hill of the right incline and distance for your workout. If the hill is not long enough, decrease the duration of the uphill sections and increase the number of reps. If you do not have access to a hill or an inclined treadmill, you can increase the resistance of the workout by running on a soft surface, such as sand or grass. Paces are difficult to translate from flat to hilly terrain, so these workouts are best done by effort (perhaps assisted by a heart rate monitor) rather than pace. For any given workout, run at the best effort you can maintain without having to slow down as the session progresses. At the end of the workout, you should feel as though you could give 10 percent more if you had to.

CROSS-TRAINING

Any sport or exercise that you do in addition to running is known as cross-training. Engaging in other forms of exercise is an effective way to perform "active recovery," which gives your body a break from the toll of running while still maintaining your fitness and adding variety to your training program.

Cross-training enables you to maintain aerobic fitness while reducing the stress of impact on your joints, muscles, and tendons. This is useful for recovery days and for rehabilitation, if you are returning to training after injury.

VARIETY AND RECOVERY

In older athletes or those with musculoskeletal conditions, cross-training helps reduce the impact on the body while maintaining training load. In younger runners, maintaining variety is important to reduce injury risk and burnout.

Multidirectional activities, such as soccer and basketball, build strength and flexibility in multiple planes and help prevent overuse injuries by adding variation to the repetitive motion of running. However, take care not to incur injuries through cross-training. Strength training (see pp.96–155) also helps prevent injury while improving performance.

RETURNING FROM INJURY

Choose types of cross-training that address your needs without aggravating your injury. For example, pool running is great when impact is the main concern; cycling or using an elliptical are other good options.

Try to mirror what you would be doing in running. For example, replace long, slow runs with long, slow pool runs or bike rides. For interval sessions, take a distance-based session (for example, 6 x 800 m) and convert it to time (for example, 6 x 3 minutes), then aim for the same intensity as the distance-based session in the pool or on the bike or elliptical. This will afford you many of the same cardiovascular benefits as running.

HOW OFTEN SHOULD I CROSS-TRAIN?

Some runners need a break from the impact of running, while others enjoy a change in routine, so the frequency of cross-training should be specific to your individual needs. In general, it is best to perform cross-training on recovery days when you do not have a key workout scheduled.

THE **TRAINING** PROGRAMS

The programs in this book each recommend three key workouts per week. Symbols are used to denote each workout type, as well as details of distance or duration, pace or effort, duration of recovery sections, and number of repetitions. Each program also includes a graph showing training volume.

THE **WORKOUTS**

All the programs (except for the Beginner 5 km walk-run program) include workouts from each of the four broad categories described on pp.180–186. In this way, all the key areas of fitness are targeted.

Longer workouts are usually easy continuous runs to develop your endurance or fast continuous runs that improve aerobic capacity, lactate clearance, and pacing. The shorter, more intense workouts are often comprised of speedwork in the form of interval training and hill training, which helps improve muscular and aerobic conditioning.

DYNAMIC WARM-UPS
Some programs prescribe a dynamic warm-up, which is a full sequence of fluid motions that is beneficial for muscle activation and injury prevention. A complete dynamic warm-up routine should consist of dynamic stretches (see pp.78–83), form drills (see pp.84–86 and p.89), and relaxed sprinting or "strides" (see p.87).

STRIDES, SPRINTS, AND ACCELERATIONS
While these are all types of short-interval training, their purpose is neurological and mechanical, as are form drills. Strides are short, fast runs that should be relaxed and performed with good form. Sprints should be high cadence, focusing on a high stride rate rather than a long stride length. Perform accelerations on the flat. Each run should gradually increase in speed to reach 100 percent intensity.

ACTIVATION SESSIONS
These sessions are designed to activate your muscles 1–2 days before a long run, hard workout, or race. The exercises used stimulate a large percentage of muscle fibers, which helps dispel sluggishness, but are short enough not to induce significant fatigue.

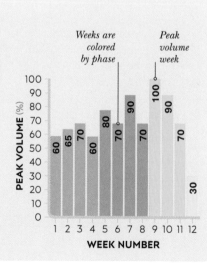

Training volume

These graphs show each program's training volume, which is measured in kilometers per week. Some programs suggest that your exercise level should be at 60 percent of the peak week before you begin. For example, if the peak volume is 100 km per week, you should be able to run 60 km per week.

If you are doing more training than the three key workouts listed, use the graph's volume percentages to scale your training, and progress gradually.

GRADUAL INCREASES
Each program increases in volume and intensity gradually to help you avoid overtraining.

Weeks are colored by phase

Peak volume week

WEEK NUMBER

PEAK VOLUME (%)

EFFORT AND PACES

For each of the workouts in the programs, there are effort or pace suggestions. Training at a range of paces broadens your running skills and improves fitness at the same time.

The suggested paces are often based on a goal distance, so to use the programs, you will need to work out your goal paces for various distances. An online pace calculator can be used to generate relatively accurate paces based on a personal best time in a race or on a realistic target time based on your current running ability. It is easiest to follow the workouts with the aid of a GPS monitor that can measure your pace during a run.

However, bear in mind that the suggested paces are targets only—maintaining good form and relaxation should be the priority. If you overreach to achieve a goal pace, you will not absorb the training load as effectively as you would have if you had run at a controlled effort. Make it your aim to finish each workout feeling like you could run 10 percent farther at the same pace if you had to.

Nondistance paces

As well as distance-based paces, the following effort-based paces are used regularly in the programs.

Easy pace should be easy enough to achieve recovery. A good guide is to set a limit of 70 percent heart rate reserve (see p.163) or to run at least 20 percent slower than your lactate threshold (LT) pace (see p.166). To calculate this, convert your LT pace to seconds and then multiply by 1.2.

Steady pace is an instruction for the recovery sections of pace-change runs. A steady pace recovery section is performed as close as possible to the pace of the fast section (ideally less than 45 sec/mile slower than the preceding fast section).

KEY TO WORKOUT SYMBOLS

Walk-run program (pp.190–191)

▪▪▪▪▪▪▪▪▪▪▪▪▪	Walk
❘❘❘❘❘❘❘❘	Run

Easy continuous runs (p.180)

• • • • • • • • • •	Short run
❘❘❘❘❘❘❘	Medium run
❘❘❘❘❘❘❘❘❘	Long run

Fast continuous runs (pp.181–183)

/❘❘❘❘❘\	Tempo run
·///////	Progression run
❘-❘-❘-❘-❘	Pace-change run

Interval training (pp.184–185)

ᴵ¹ᴵ¹ᴵ¹ᴵ¹ᴵ¹	Strides
₁❘₁❘₁❘₁❘₁	Sprints
ₐₗ❘ₗₐₗ❘ₗₐₗ❘	Accelerations
•❘❘•❘❘•❘❘•	Anaerobic capacity training
•❘❘❘❘❘❘❘	VO₂ max training

Hill training (p.186)

↗↗↗	Hill run

Other

 Dynamic warm-up

Pace and effort notations

E	Easy pace (RPE 2)
S	Steady pace
LT	Lactate threshold pace (RPE 4.3)
MP	Marathon pace
HMP	Half marathon pace
10km	10-km pace
5km	5-km pace
3km	3-km pace
1500m	1500-m pace
800m	800-m pace
VO₂	VO₂ max effort (RPE 6–7)
AC	Anaerobic capacity effort (RPE 8–9)
100i	100 percent intensity (RPE 10)
○	Recovery walk/jog half the duration of the run
●	Recovery walk/jog equal to the duration of the run
●●	Recovery walk/jog twice the duration of the run
●●●●	Recovery walk/jog four times the duration of the run

Shorthand symbols

⋈	Alternate between paces	>	Run faster than given pace
↑	Uphill run/walk/jog	<	Run slower than given pace
↓	Downhill run/walk/jog	@	Run at a given pace
⌐ x 4 ⌐	Number of repetitions		

BEGINNER 5 KM PROGRAM

If you are completely new to running, this walk-run program will build your capacity to run from 1 minute at a time to 30 minutes continuously within 12 weeks. Those returning to training after injury can also use this program but may be able to progress more quickly, or start at a later week. Plan your return to running with a physical therapist so your progress can be monitored.

PROGRAM GOALS

This program aims to help you achieve a target distance of 5 km. Running continuously for 30 minutes will cover 5 km if your pace is 6:00 min/km or faster. If it is slower than this, you can achieve 5 km by extending the program. For example, if your pace is 7:00 min/km, aim for a run of 35 minutes. In addition, you could extend the duration of your workout by performing for an extra 10 minutes.

Begin each session with 5 minutes of walking to warm up. Perform the run sections at easy pace (easy enough to carry a conversation while you are running). Do not hesitate to repeat a workout or a week if you do not feel ready for the next level. Take at least 1 day of rest, or do cross-training, between each walk-run workout.

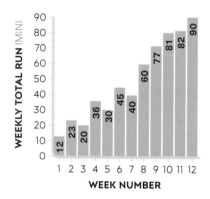

TOTAL RUN TIME PER WEEK
This graph shows how the total time you will be running (versus walking) builds up over the 12-week program.

> **FOR KEY TO WORKOUT SYMBOLS
> SEE PP.188–189**

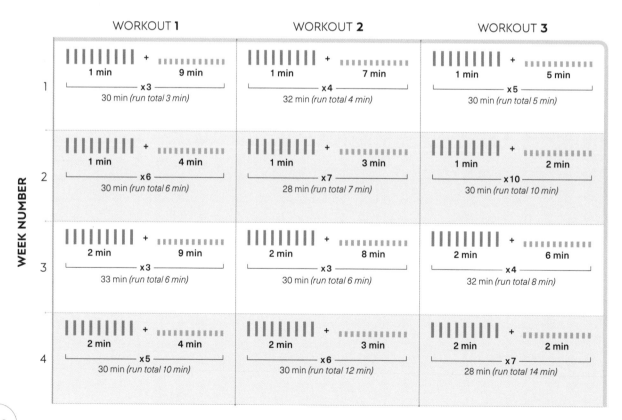

	WORKOUT 1	WORKOUT 2	WORKOUT 3
5	3 min + 7 min — x3 — 30 min *(run total 9 min)*	3 min + 6 min — x3 — 27 min *(run total 9 min)*	3 min + 5 min — x4 — 32 min *(run total 12 min)*
6	3 min + 4 min — x4 — 28 min *(run total 12 min)*	3 min + 3 min — x5 — 30 min *(run total 15 min)*	3 min + 2 min — x6 — 30 min *(run total 18 min)*
7	4 min + 6 min — x3 — 30 min *(run total 12 min)*	4 min + 5 min — x3 — 27 min *(run total 12 min)*	4 min + 4 min — x4 — 32 min *(run total 16 min)*
8	4 min + 3 min — x4 — 28 min *(run total 16 min)*	4 min + 2 min — x5 — 30 min *(run total 20 min)*	4 min + 1 min — x6 — 30 min *(run total 24 min)*
9	5 min + 1 min — x5 — 30 min *(run total 25 min)*	6 min + 1 min — x4 — 28 min *(run total 24 min)*	7 min + 1 min — x4 — 32 min *(run total 28 min)*
10	8 min + 1 min — x3 — 27 min *(run total 24 min)*	9 min + 1 min — x3 — 30 min *(run total 27 min)*	10 min + 1 min — x3 — 33 min *(run total 30 min)*
11	12 min + 1 min — x2 — 26 min *(run total 24 min)*	14 min + 1 min — x2 — 30 min *(run total 28 min)*	18 min + 1 min + 12 min — x1 — 31 min *(run total 30 min)*
12	20 min + 1 min + 10 min — x1 — 31 min *(run total 30 min)*	24 min + 1 min + 6 min — x1 — 31 min *(run total 30 min)*	30 min

WEEK NUMBER

191

BEGINNER 10 KM PROGRAM

This program prepares you to complete 10 km in your first race. Before starting, you should be capable of a continuous 3-mile run, be running 3 times a week, and have built up an exercise volume equivalent to 60 percent of the program's peak volume.

In this program, any workout beginning with a pace other than easy should be preceded by a 10-minute easy run and a dynamic warm-up.

PROGRAM GOALS

Weeks 1–4 focus on base-building by increasing the distance of the long run. Perform the 30-second stride workouts in a form-focused but relaxed way, to create an easy, efficient stride. Recover in week 4.

In the support phase, the program intensifies with pace-change runs, interval training, and hill training. Like the strides, the hill reps should be done with form and relaxation as the main goals. Week 8 is a recovery week, with easier workouts and a shorter long run.

Weeks 9–12 are race-specific, with longer pace-change and intervals workouts. During the taper in week 12, reduce any easy runs or cross-training to less than 50 percent of your usual volume.

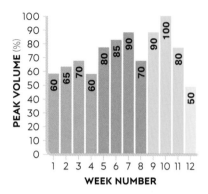

TRAINING VOLUME PER WEEK
The training volume builds gradually, peaking in week 10. Weeks 4 and 8 are recovery weeks, and week 12 is tapered.

> **FOR KEY TO WORKOUT SYMBOLS SEE PP.188–189**

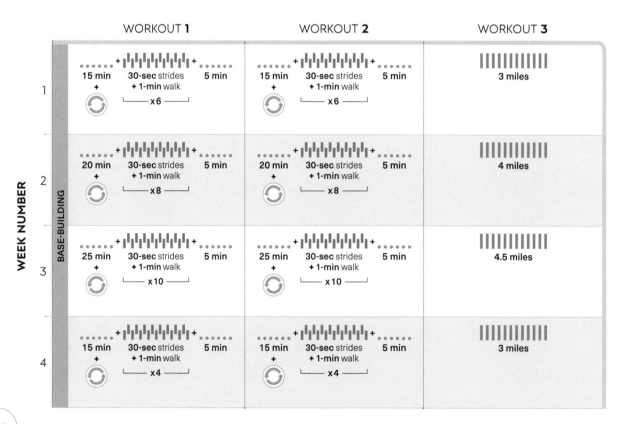

	WORKOUT **1**	WORKOUT **2**	WORKOUT **3**

WEEK NUMBER

SUPPORT

Week 5

Workout 1: 15 min — 1 min @ LT with 4 min @ E, end with 5-min walk + 30-sec strides + 1-min walk — x4

Workout 2: 2 miles + — ↑30-sec run @ AC + ↓90-sec walk — x6

Workout 3: 4.5 miles — *Finish the last* **half mile** *@* LT *if you are feeling strong*

Week 6

Workout 1: 18 min — 2 min @ LT with 4 min @ E, end with 5-min walk + 30-sec strides + 1-min walk — x4

Workout 2: 1 min @ 3km + 1-min walk — x10

Workout 3: 5 miles — *Finish the last* **half mile** *@* LT *if you are feeling strong*

Week 7

Workout 1: 24 min — 4 min @ LT with 4 min @ E, end with 5-min walk + 30-sec strides + 1-min walk — x4

Workout 2: 2.5 miles + — ↑30-sec run @ AC + ↓90-sec walk — x8

Workout 3: 5 miles — *Finish the last* **mile** *@* LT *if you are feeling strong*

Week 8

Workout 1: 15 min — 1 min @ LT with 4 min @ E, end with 5-min walk + 30-sec strides + 1-min walk — x4

Workout 2: 15 min + 30-sec strides + 1-min walk 5 min — x6

Workout 3: 4 miles

RACE-SPECIFIC

Week 9

Workout 1: 24 min — 6 min @ LT with 2 min @ E, end with 5-min walk + 30-sec strides + 1-min walk — x4

Workout 2: 3 min @ 5km + 90-sec walk — x6

Workout 3: 5.5 miles — *Finish the last* **1.5 miles** *@* LT *if you are feeling strong*

Week 10

Workout 1: 20 min — 8 min @ LT with 2 min @ E, end with 5-min walk + 30-sec strides + 1-min walk — x4

Workout 2: 2.5 miles + — ↑30-sec run @ AC + ↓90-sec walk — x10

Workout 3: 5.5 miles — *Finish the last* **2 miles** *@* LT *if you are feeling strong*

Week 11

Workout 1: 20 min @ LT, end with 5-min walk + 30-sec strides + 1-min walk — x4

Workout 2: 4 min @ 5km + 2-min walk — x3 + 2 min @ 3km + 2-min walk — x3

Workout 3: 4 miles

TAPER

Week 12

Workout 1: 15 min — 1 min @ LT with 4 min @ E, end with 5-min walk + 30-sec strides + 1-min walk — x4

Workout 2: 15 min + 30-sec strides + 1-min walk 5 min — x6 — *2–3 days before race*

Workout 3: **RACE DAY**

ADVANCED 10 KM PROGRAM

If you have competed in 10 km races before, this program is designed to help you improve your race times by building up the intensity and duration of the workouts. You should be able to run continuously for 10 miles before starting this program.

In this program, any workout that begins with marathon pace or faster (see pp.188–189) should be preceded by a 2-mile easy run and a dynamic warm-up.

INTRODUCTION PHASE

This phase prepares you for the base-building phase by building up to 60 percent of peak volume. This may take longer than three weeks, depending on your starting point, so repeat a week if needed.

BASE-BUILDING PHASE

Weeks 4–9 will raise aerobic volume, introduce aerobic intensity, and improve your running skills. Workout 1 focuses on interval training on hills and on the flat.

Workout 2 consists of short and medium fast continuous runs with increasing intensity, while the long runs of workout 3 increase in volume and aerobic intensity.

SUPPORT PHASE

In week 10, workouts 1 and 2 are lighter to aid recovery. Weeks 11–15 continue to increase aerobic volume and aim to improve your speed endurance, lactate threshold speed, and ability to clear lactate. In workout 1, the short and medium runs become more difficult, and longer hill workouts at VO2 max effort are added. Workout 2 introduces VO2 max and anaerobic-capacity intervals. Workout 3 expands the time spent at half marathon pace (HMP) and increases the pace of the steady recoveries during these runs.

RACE-SPECIFIC PHASE

Following lighter workouts in week 16 to aid recovery, weeks 17–24 prepare you to run at goal race pace and keep lactate levels relatively low so that your muscles can clear any accumulated lactate quickly. Workouts 1 and 2 consist of pace-change runs at 10 km, fast continuous runs that increase in duration, short-hill sprints to maintain power, and interval training to maintain speed. For workout 3, during pace-change runs at HMP, keep the steady pace sections as close to HMP as possible.

TAPER

The 13-day taper in weeks 23 and 24 is divided into 3 parts: an initial 5-day taper kick-starts your recovery after the peak training phase; the next 4 days increase the load slightly to include workouts that maintain your fitness without stressing your body; and a final 4-day taper during which you should perform only an activation session before your race.

> **FOR KEY TO WORKOUT SYMBOLS SEE PP.188–189**

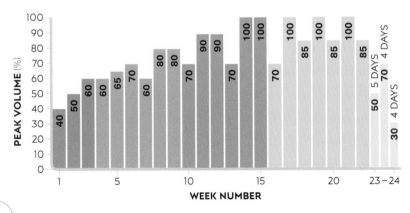

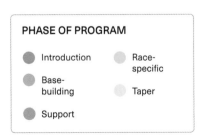

PHASE OF PROGRAM

- Introduction
- Base-building
- Support
- Race-specific
- Taper

TRAINING VOLUME PER WEEK
Training volume peaks in week 14 and is maintained (not increased) until a 13-day taper, which is split into 3 parts.

	WORKOUT **1**	WORKOUT **2**	WORKOUT **3**
1	30 min	30 min	6 miles
2	40 min + ↻	40 min + ↻	7.5 miles
3	50 min + ↻	50 min + ↻	9 miles
4	30-sec sprint + 60–90-sec walk — x8	30 min ⋈ 1 min @ 15 sec > LT with 2 min @ E	9 miles ⋈ 7.5 miles @ E with 1.5 miles @ HMP
5	↑10-sec run @ 100i, +↓2-min walk — x5 + 30-sec sprint + 60–90-sec walk — x5	30 min 10 min @ 60 sec < LT + 8 min @ 45 sec < LT + 6 min @ 30 sec < LT + 4 min @ 15 sec < LT + 2 min @ LT	10 miles ⋈ 2.5 miles @ E with 0.5 miles @ LT
6	↑10-sec run @ 100i, +↓2-min walk — x8 + 30-sec sprint + 60–90-sec walk — x4	50 min 30 min @ E + 10 min @ LT + 10 min @ E	5 x 2-mile runs @ 90 sec < HMP + @ 75 sec < HMP + @ 50 sec < HMP + @ 25 sec < HMP + @ HMP
7	↑15-sec run @ 100i, +↓2-min walk — x8 + 30-sec accelerations + 60–90-sec walk — x4	30 min ⋈ 90 sec @ 15 sec > LT with 90 sec @ E	12 miles 4 miles @ E + 4 miles @ MP + 4 miles @ E
8	↑15-sec run @ 100i, +↓2-min walk — x10 + 30-sec accelerations + 60–90-sec walk — x4	5 x 6-min runs @ 60 sec < LT + @ 45 sec < LT + @ 30 sec < LT + @ 15 sec < LT + @ LT	2 miles + 10 miles ⋈ 0.5 miles @ LT with 1.5 miles @ E

WEEK NUMBER

INTRODUCTION (weeks 1–3) · BASE-BUILDING (weeks 4–8)

ADVANCED 10 KM

	WORKOUT 1	WORKOUT 2	WORKOUT 3
BASE-BUILDING 9	↑ 15-sec run @ 100i, + ↓ 2-min walk — x10 — + 30-sec accelerations + 60–90-sec walk — x6 —	50 min 20 min @ E + 20 min @ LT + 10 min @ E	4 x 3-mile runs @ 90 sec < MP + @ 60 sec < MP + @ 30 sec < MP + @ MP
10	30 min ⤄ 4 min @ LT with 2 min @ E, end with 5-min walk + 30 sec @ 3km – 1500m, 1-min walk — x4 —	20–30 min + ↻ (ACTIVATION) + ↑ 10-sec run @ 100i, + ↓ 2-min walk — x4 —	9 miles 3 miles @ E + 3 miles @ HMP + 3 miles @ E _or substitute with a 3–5 km race_
11	↑ 15-sec run @ 100i, + ↓ 2-min walk — x4 — + ↑ 1-min run @ VO₂, + ↓ 2-min jog — x12 —	300m @ 1500m + ●● walk/jog — x5 — + 200m @ 800m + ●●●● walk/jog — x5 —	2 miles + 12 miles ⤄ 0.5 miles @ LT with 1 mile @ E
SUPPORT 12	↑ 15-sec run @ 100i, + ↓ 2-min walk — x4 — + 21 min ⤄ 1 min @ 15 sec > LT with 2 min @ S	800m @ 3km + ● walk/jog — x5 — + 200m @ 1500m + ●● walk/jog — x4 —	5 x 2-mile runs @ 60 sec < HMP + @ 45 sec < HMP + @ 30 sec < HMP + @ 15 sec < HMP + @ HMP
13	↑ 15-sec run @ 100i, + ↓ 2-min walk — x4 — + ↑ 90-sec run @ VO₂, + ↓ 3-min jog — x8 —	400m @ 1500m + ●● walk/jog — x5 — + 200m @ 800m + ●●●● walk/jog — x5 —	14 miles 3 miles @ E + 8 miles @ MP + 3 miles @ E
14	↑ 15-sec run @ 100i, + ↓ 2-min walk — x4 — + 4 x 6-min runs + @ 45 sec < LT + @ 30 sec < LT + @ 15 sec < LT + @ LT	1000m @ 3km + ● walk/jog — x4 — + 200m @ 1500m + ●● walk/jog — x4 —	10 miles ⤄ 1.5 mile @ LT with 0.5 miles @ E
15	↑ 15-sec run @ 100i, + ↓ 2-min walk — x4 — + ↑ 2-min run @ VO₂, + ↓ 2-min jog — x6 —	600m @ 1500m + ●● walk/jog — x4 — + 200m @ 800m + ●●●● walk/jog — x5 —	4 x 4-mile runs @ 75 sec < MP + @ 50 sec < MP + @ 25 sec < MP + @ MP
RACE-SPECIFIC 16	30 min ⤄ 4 min @ LT with 2 min @ E end with 5-min walk + 30 sec @ 3km + 1-min walk — x4 —	20–30 min + ↻ (ACTIVATION) + ↑ 10-sec run @ 100i, + ↓ 2-min walk — x4 —	10 miles 2.5 miles @ E + 5 miles @ HMP + 2.5 miles @ E _or substitute with a 5–8 km race_

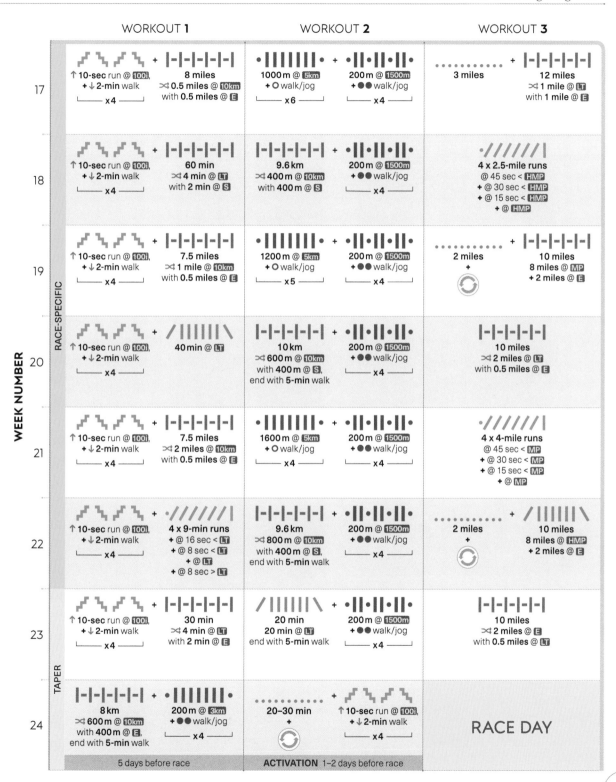

	WORKOUT **1**	WORKOUT **2**	WORKOUT **3**
17	↑ 10-sec run @ 100i, + ↓ 2-min walk ⎿ x4 ⏋ + 8 miles ⊃⊲ 0.5 miles @ 10km with 0.5 miles @ E	1000 m @ 5km + ○ walk/jog ⎿ x6 ⏋ + 200 m @ 1500m + ●● walk/jog ⎿ x4 ⏋	3 miles + 12 miles ⊃⊲ 1 mile @ LT with 1 mile @ E
18	↑ 10-sec run @ 100i, + ↓ 2-min walk ⎿ x4 ⏋ + 60 min ⊃⊲ 4 min @ LT with 2 min @ S	9.6 km ⊃⊲ 400 m @ 10km with 400 m @ S + 200 m @ 1500m + ●● walk/jog ⎿ x4 ⏋	4 x 2.5-mile runs @ 45 sec < HMP + @ 30 sec < HMP + @ 15 sec < HMP + @ HMP
19	↑ 10-sec run @ 100i, + ↓ 2-min walk ⎿ x4 ⏋ + 7.5 miles ⊃⊲ 1 mile @ 10km with 0.5 miles @ E	1200 m @ 5km + ○ walk/jog ⎿ x5 ⏋ + 200 m @ 1500m + ●● walk/jog ⎿ x4 ⏋	2 miles + ⟲ 10 miles 8 miles @ MP + 2 miles @ E
20	↑ 10-sec run @ 100i, + ↓ 2-min walk ⎿ x4 ⏋ + 40 min @ LT	10 km ⊃⊲ 600 m @ 10km with 400 m @ S, end with 5-min walk + 200 m @ 1500m + ●● walk/jog ⎿ x4 ⏋	10 miles ⊃⊲ 2 miles @ LT with 0.5 miles @ E
21	↑ 10-sec run @ 100i, + ↓ 2-min walk ⎿ x4 ⏋ + 7.5 miles ⊃⊲ 2 miles @ 10km with 0.5 miles @ E	1600 m @ 5km + ○ walk/jog ⎿ x4 ⏋ + 200 m @ 1500m + ●● walk/jog ⎿ x4 ⏋	4 x 4-mile runs @ 45 sec < MP + @ 30 sec < MP + @ 15 sec < MP + @ MP
22	↑ 10-sec run @ 100i, + ↓ 2-min walk ⎿ x4 ⏋ + 4 x 9-min runs + @ 16 sec < LT + @ 8 sec < LT + @ LT + @ 8 sec > LT	9.6 km ⊃⊲ 800 m @ 10km with 400 m @ S, end with 5-min walk + 200 m @ 1500m + ●● walk/jog ⎿ x4 ⏋	2 miles + ⟲ 10 miles 8 miles @ HMP + 2 miles @ E
23	↑ 10-sec run @ 100i, + ↓ 2-min walk ⎿ x4 ⏋ + 30 min ⊃⊲ 4 min @ LT with 2 min @ E	20 min 20 min @ LT end with 5-min walk + 200 m @ 1500m + ●● walk/jog ⎿ x4 ⏋	10 miles ⊃⊲ 2 miles @ E with 0.5 miles @ LT
24	8 km ⊃⊲ 600 m @ 10km with 400 m @ E, end with 5-min walk + 200 m @ 3km + ●● walk/jog ⎿ x4 ⏋	20–30 min + ⟲ + ↑ 10-sec run @ 100i, + ↓ 2-min walk ⎿ x4 ⏋	**RACE DAY**
	5 days before race	**ACTIVATION** 1–2 days before race	

WEEK NUMBER

RACE-SPECIFIC (weeks 17–22)

TAPER (weeks 23–24)

BEGINNER HALF MARATHON PROGRAM

This program trains you to complete a first half marathon. Before starting, you should be capable of a continuous 6-mile run, be running 3 times a week, and have built up an exercise volume equivalent to 60 percent of the program's peak volume.

In this program, any workout starting faster than easy pace should be preceded by a 10-minute easy run and a dynamic warm-up.

PROGRAM GOALS

During base-building in weeks 1–4, the aims are to build volume via long runs, introduce intensity with

short and long pace-change runs, and improve form with strides, sprints, and hill workouts.

Weeks 5–8 (support phase) introduce interval training at 3 km pace and 1500 m pace. Easy continuous runs are longer, and the ratio of fast to easy pace running becomes harder.

Weeks 9–12 are race-specific. The long runs and fast continuous runs both become longer and the ratio of fast to easy pace running increases. Interval training shifts to 5 km pace. Begin the 7–8-day taper in week 12 the weekend before your race, after the long run in week 11.

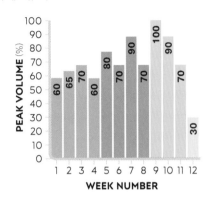

TRAINING VOLUME PER WEEK
The training volume builds to a peak in week 9. Week 12 drops to 30 percent volume, so you are fresh for your race.

**FOR KEY TO WORKOUT SYMBOLS
SEE PP.188–189**

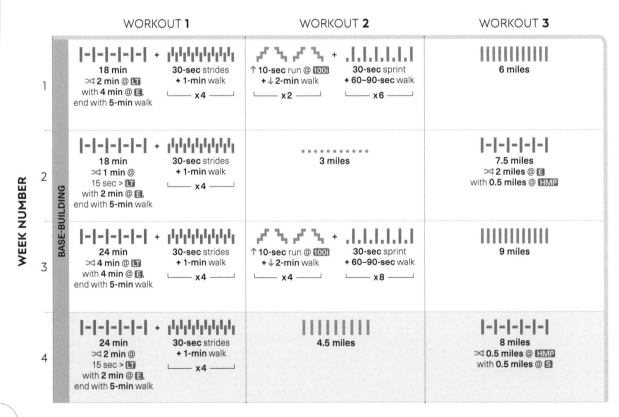

WORKOUT **1** | WORKOUT **2** | WORKOUT **3**

Week 1
18 min — 2 min @ LT with 4 min @ E, end with 5-min walk + 30-sec strides + 1-min walk x4 | ↑10-sec run @ 100i + ↓2-min walk x2 + 30-sec sprint + 60–90-sec walk x6 | 6 miles

Week 2
18 min — 1 min @ 15 sec > LT with 2 min @ E, end with 5-min walk + 30-sec strides + 1-min walk x4 | 3 miles | 7.5 miles — 2 miles @ E with 0.5 miles @ HMP

Week 3
24 min — 4 min @ LT with 4 min @ E, end with 5-min walk + 30-sec strides + 1-min walk x4 | ↑10-sec run @ 100i + ↓2-min walk x4 + 30-sec sprint + 60–90-sec walk x8 | 9 miles

Week 4
24 min — 2 min @ 15 sec > LT with 2 min @ E, end with 5-min walk + 30-sec strides + 1-min walk x4 | 4.5 miles | 8 miles — 0.5 miles @ HMP with 0.5 miles @ S

BASE-BUILDING

WEEK NUMBER

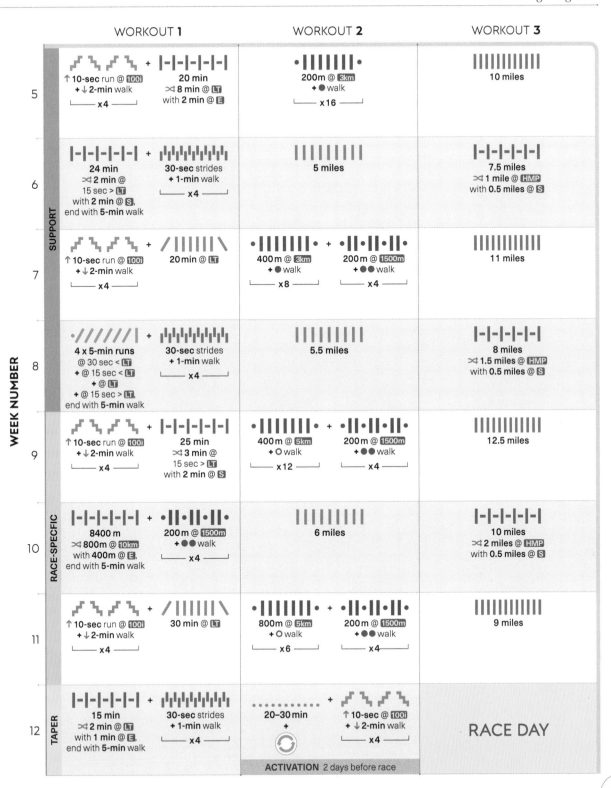

WORKOUT **1** WORKOUT **2** WORKOUT **3**

WEEK NUMBER

SUPPORT

5

↑ 10-sec run @ 100j + ↓ 2-min walk — x4

20 min ✂ 8 min @ LT with 2 min @ E

200m @ 3km + ● walk — x16

10 miles

6

24 min ✂ 2 min @ 15 sec > LT with 2 min @ S, end with 5-min walk

30-sec strides + 1-min walk — x4

5 miles

7.5 miles ✂ 1 mile @ HMP with 0.5 miles @ S

7

↑ 10-sec run @ 100j + ↓ 2-min walk — x4

20 min @ LT

400m @ 3km + ● walk — x8

200m @ 1500m + ●● walk — x4

11 miles

8

4 x 5-min runs @ 30 sec < LT + 15 sec < LT + @ LT + @ 15 sec > LT, end with 5-min walk

30-sec strides + 1-min walk — x4

5.5 miles

8 miles ✂ 1.5 miles @ HMP with 0.5 miles @ S

9

↑ 10-sec run @ 100j + ↓ 2-min walk — x4

25 min ✂ 3 min @ 15 sec > LT with 2 min @ S

400m @ 5km + ○ walk — x12

200m @ 1500m + ●● walk — x4

12.5 miles

RACE-SPECIFIC

10

8400 m ✂ 800m @ 10km with 400m @ E, end with 5-min walk

200m @ 1500m + ●● walk — x4

6 miles

10 miles ✂ 2 miles @ HMP with 0.5 miles @ S

11

↑ 10-sec run @ 100j + ↓ 2-min walk — x4

30 min @ LT

800m @ 5km + ○ walk — x6

200m @ 1500m + ●● walk — x4

9 miles

TAPER

12

15 min ✂ 2 min @ LT with 1 min @ E, end with 5-min walk

30-sec strides + 1-min walk — x4

20–30 min + ↻

↑ 10-sec @ 100j + ↓ 2-min walk — x4

RACE DAY

ACTIVATION 2 days before race

199

ADVANCED HALF MARATHON PROGRAM

This program is ideal when you have completed a major race and want to prepare for the next half marathon. Over 24 weeks, this training program aims to help you reach your goal race time.

In this program, any workout that begins with marathon pace or faster (see pp.188–189) should be preceded by a 2-mile easy run and a dynamic warm-up.

INTRODUCTION PHASE

Your goal in this phase is to recover from the previous race and achieve 60 percent of peak training volume before starting the next phase. This may take longer than three weeks, so repeat a week if needed.

BASE-BUILDING PHASE

In weeks 4–9, workout 1 improves running skills with short sprints (on hills and on the flat); workout 2 introduces aerobic intensity with short and medium fast continuous runs; and workout 3 builds aerobic volume and intensity with long fast continuous runs.

SUPPORT PHASE

Recover in week 10 with lighter sessions for workouts 1 and 2. Weeks 11–15 aim to improve your aerobic volume, speed endurance, lactate threshold speed, and lactate clearance. For workout 1, the pace-change and progression runs become harder, and longer hill workouts are introduced. Workout 2 introduces VO₂ max and anaerobic capacity intervals. The long runs for workout 3 are designed to help you practice half marathon goal pace.

RACE-SPECIFIC PHASE

Lighter workouts in week 16 will help you recover before weeks 17–22, during which you will spend longer running at goal race pace. Workout 1 increases the difficulty of the pace-change runs to improve your ability to clear lactate from the muscles and includes short sprints to maintain power. Workout 2 contains short-hill sprints and medium fast continuous runs that increase in intensity. Workout 3 focuses on long runs at half marathon pace (HMP); aim to keep the steady pace sections of these runs as close to HMP as possible.

TAPER

The 13-day taper in weeks 23 and 24 is divided into 3 parts: an initial 5-day taper kick-starts your recovery after training at peak volume in weeks 20–22; the next 4 days increase the load slightly to include workouts that maintain your fitness without stressing your body; and a final 4-day taper during which you should perform only an activation session before your race.

**FOR KEY TO WORKOUT SYMBOLS
SEE PP.188–189**

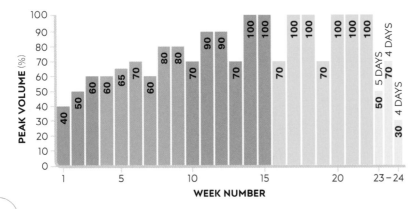

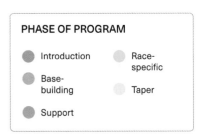

PHASE OF PROGRAM

- Introduction
- Base-building
- Support
- Race-specific
- Taper

TRAINING VOLUME PER WEEK
Training volume peaks in week 14 and is maintained (not increased) until a 13-day taper, which is split into 3 parts.

	WORKOUT **1**	WORKOUT **2**	WORKOUT **3**

WEEK NUMBER

INTRODUCTION

1

Workout 1: 30 min

Workout 2: 30 min

Workout 3: 6 miles

2

Workout 1: 40 min +

Workout 2: 40 min +

Workout 3: 7.5 miles

3

Workout 1: 50 min +

Workout 2: 50 min +

Workout 3: 9 miles

BASE-BUILDING

4

Workout 1: 30-sec sprint + 60–90-sec walk — x8 —

Workout 2: 30 min ⊃⊂ 1 min @ 15 sec > **LT** with 2 min @ **E**

Workout 3: 3 miles + 6 miles ⊃⊂ 0.5 miles @ **LT** with 1 mile @ **E**

5

Workout 1: ↑10-sec run @ **100i** + ↓2-min walk — x5 — + 30-sec sprint + 60–90-sec walk — x5 —

Workout 2: 50 min 30 min @ **E** + 10 min @ **LT** + 10 min @ **E**

Workout 3: 4 x 2.5-mile runs @ 1 min 40 sec < **HMP** + @ 1 min 15 sec < **HMP** + @ 50 sec < **HMP** + @ 25 sec < **HMP**

6

Workout 1: ↑10-sec run @ **100i** + ↓2-min walk — x8 — + 30-sec sprint + 60–90-sec walk — x4 —

Workout 2: 30 min 10 min @ 60 sec < **LT** + 8 min @ 45 sec < **LT** + 6 min @ 30 sec < **LT** + 4 min @ 15 sec < **LT** + 2 min @ **LT**

Workout 3: 2.5 miles + 7.5 miles ⊃⊂ 2 miles @ 30 sec < **HMP** with 0.5 miles @ **E**

7

Workout 1: ↑15-sec run @ **100i** + ↓2-min walk — x8 — + 30-sec accelerations + 60–90-sec walk — x4 —

Workout 2: 30 min ⊃⊂ 90 sec @ 15 sec > **LT** with 90 sec @ **E**

Workout 3: 2 miles + 8 miles ⊃⊂ 0.5 miles @ **LT** with 0.5 miles @ **E**

8

Workout 1: ↑15-sec run @ **100i** + ↓2-min walk — x10 — + 30-sec accelerations + 60–90-sec walk — x4 —

Workout 2: 50 min 20 min @ **E** + 20 min @ **LT** + 10 min @ **E**

Workout 3: 6 x 2-mile runs @ 90 sec < **HMP** + @ 75 sec < **HMP** + @ 60 sec < **HMP** + @ 45 sec < **HMP** + @ 30 sec < **HMP** + @ 15 sec < **HMP**

HALF MARATHON
ADVANCED

WEEK NUMBER

	WORKOUT 1	WORKOUT 2	WORKOUT 3
9 (BASE-BUILDING)	↑15-sec run @ 100i +↓2-min walk — x10 + 30-sec accelerations + 60–90-sec walk — x6	5 x 6-min runs @ 60 sec < LT + @ 45 sec < LT + @ 30 sec < LT + @ 15 sec < LT + @ LT	2 miles + 10 miles ⤢ 2 miles @ 30 sec < HMP with 0.5 miles @ E
10	30 min ⤢ 4 min @ LT with 2 min @ E, end with 5-min walk + 30 sec @ 3km – 1500m + 1-min walk — x4	20–30 min + ↻ + ↑10-sec run @ 100i +↓2-min walk — x4 **ACTIVATION**	8 miles ⤢ 0.5 miles @ HMP with 0.5 miles @ S *or substitute with a 5–8 km race*
11	↑15-sec run @ 100i +↓2-min walk — x4 + ↑1-min run @ VO₂ +↓2-min jog — x12	1000m @ 5km + ○ walk/jog — x6 + 200 m @ 1500m + ●● walk/jog — x4	12 miles 2 miles @ E + 8 miles @ 30 sec < HMP + 2 miles @ E
12 (SUPPORT)	↑15-sec run @ 100i +↓2-min walk — x4 + 20 min ⤢ 1 min @ 15 sec > LT with 2 min @ S, end with 5-min walk	800m @ 3km + ● walk/jog — x5 + 200 m @ 1500m + ●● walk/jog — x4	5 x 2.5-mile runs @ 1 min 40 sec < HMP + @ 1 min 15 sec < HMP + @ 50 sec < HMP + @ 25 sec < HMP + @ HMP
13	↑15-sec run @ 100i +↓2-min walk — x4 + ↑90-sec run @ VO₂ +↓3-min jog — x8	1200m @ 5km + ○ walk/jog — x5 + 200 m @ 1500m + ●● walk/jog — x4	9 miles ⤢ 1 mile @ HMP with 0.5 miles @ S
14	↑15-sec run @ 100i +↓2-min walk — x4 + 4 x 6-min runs @ 45 sec < LT + @ 30 sec < LT + @ 15 sec < LT + @ LT	1000m @ 3km + ● walk/jog — x4 + 200 m @ 1500m + ●● walk/jog — x4	14 miles 2 miles @ E + 10 miles @ 25 sec < HMP + 2 miles @ E
15	↑15-sec run @ 100i +↓2-min walk — x4 + ↑2-min run @ VO₂ +↓4-min jog — x6	1600m @ 5km + ○ walk/jog — x4 + 200 m @ 1500m + ●● walk/jog — x4	4 x 3-mile runs @ 75 sec < HMP + @ 50 sec < HMP + @ 25 sec < HMP + @ HMP
16 (RACE-SPECIFIC)	30 min ⤢ 4 min @ LT with 2 min @ E, end with 5-min walk + 30 sec @ 3km + 1-min walk — x4	20–30 min + ↻ + ↑10-sec run @ 100i +↓2-min walk — x4 **ACTIVATION**	10 miles ⤢ 1.5 miles @ HMP with 0.5 miles @ S *or substitute with a 10–15 km race*

	WORKOUT **1**	WORKOUT **2**	WORKOUT **3**
17 (RACE-SPECIFIC)	30 min ⤫ 2 min @ 15 sec > LT with 3 min @ S, end with 5-min walk **+** 30 sec @ 3km – 1500m + 1-min walk ×6	↑ 10-sec run @ 100i + ↓ 2-min walk ×4 **+** 60 min ⤫ 3 min @ LT with 3 min @ S	2.5 miles **+** (optional) ↻ **+** 12.5 miles 10 miles @ 15 sec < HMP + 2.5 miles @ E
18	8 miles ⤫ 0.5 miles @ 10km with 0.5 miles @ E, end with 5-min walk **+** 30 sec @ 3km – 1500m + 1-min walk ×6	↑ 10-sec run @ 100i + ↓ 2-min walk ×4 **+** 35 min @ LT	5 × 3-mile runs @ 80 sec < HMP + @ 60 sec < HMP + @ 40 sec < HMP + @ 20 sec < HMP + @ HMP
19	30 min ⤫ 3 min @ 15 sec > LT with 3 min @ S, end with 5-min walk **+** 30 sec @ 3km – 1500m + 1-min walk ×6	↑ 10-sec run @ 100i + ↓ 2-min walk ×4 **+** 4 × 9-min runs @ 24 sec < LT + @ 16 sec < LT + @ 8 sec < LT + @ LT	10 miles ⤫ 2 miles @ HMP with 0.5 miles @ S
20	7.5 miles ⤫ 1 mile @ 10km with 0.5 miles @ E, end with 5-min walk **+** 30 sec @ 3km – 1500m + 1-min walk ×6	↑ 10-sec run @ 100i + ↓ 2-min walk ×4 **+** 60 min ⤫ 4 min @ LT with 2 min @ S	2.5 miles **+** (optional) ↻ **+** 12.5 miles 10 miles @ 10 sec < HMP + 2.5 miles @ E
21	30 min ⤫ 3 min @ 15 sec > LT with 2 min @ S, end with 5-min walk **+** 30 sec @ 3km – 1500m + 1-min walk ×6	↑ 10-sec run @ 100i + ↓ 2-min walk ×4 **+** 40 min @ LT	5 × 3-mile runs @ 45 sec < HMP + @ 35 sec < HMP + @ 25 sec < HMP + @ 15 sec < HMP + @ HMP
22	7.5 miles ⤫ 2 miles @ 10km with 0.5 miles @ E, end with 5-min walk **+** 30 sec @ 3km – 1500m + 1-min walk ×6	↑ 10-sec run @ 100i + ↓ 2-min walk ×4 **+** 4 × 9-min runs @ 16 sec < LT + @ 8 sec < LT + @ LT + 8 sec > LT	9 miles @ HMP
23 (TAPER)	30 min ⤫ 4 min @ LT with 2 min @ E, end with 5-min walk **+** 30 sec @ 3km – 1500m + 1-min walk ×4	↑ 10-sec run @ 100i + ↓ 2-min walk ×4 **+** 20 min @ LT	10 miles ⤫ 2 miles @ E with 0.5 miles @ HMP
24	5 miles ⤫ 0.5 miles @ HMP with 0.5 miles @ E, end with 5-min walk **+** 30 sec @ 3km + 1-min walk ×6	20–30 min **+** ↻	**+** ↑ 10-sec run @ 100i + ↓ 2-min walk ×4	RACE DAY
	5 days before race	**ACTIVATION** 1 or 2 days before race	

BEGINNER MARATHON PROGRAM

This program prepares you for a first marathon. Before starting, you should be capable of running 13 miles continuously, be running at least 3 times a week, and have built up an exercise volume equivalent to 60 percent of the program's peak volume.

In this program, any workout beginning with a pace other than easy should be preceded by a 10-minute easy run and a dynamic warm-up.

PROGRAM GOALS

During base-building, weeks 1–4, long runs increase in intensity and distance, while strides, sprints, and hill training are introduced to improve speed and power.

In weeks 5–8, the support phase introduces anaerobic capacity and VO₂ max intervals to improve lactate clearance. The volume of fast continuous and long runs increases to help improve your endurance.

The race-specific phase, weeks 9–12, focuses on aerobic intensity, with workouts ranging from marathon pace to slightly faster than lactate threshold pace. Allowing time for rest and recovery before the race are the main goals in the final three weeks.

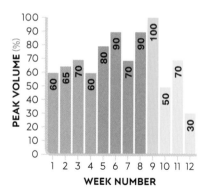

TRAINING VOLUME PER WEEK
The training volume builds gradually to a peak in week 9. A long taper period allows adequate recovery before racing.

> **FOR KEY TO WORKOUT SYMBOLS
> SEE PP.188–189**

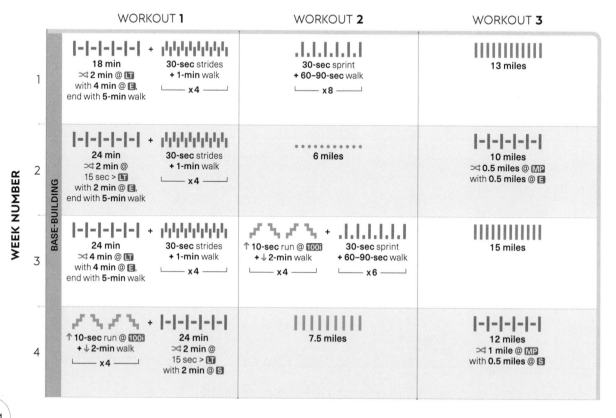

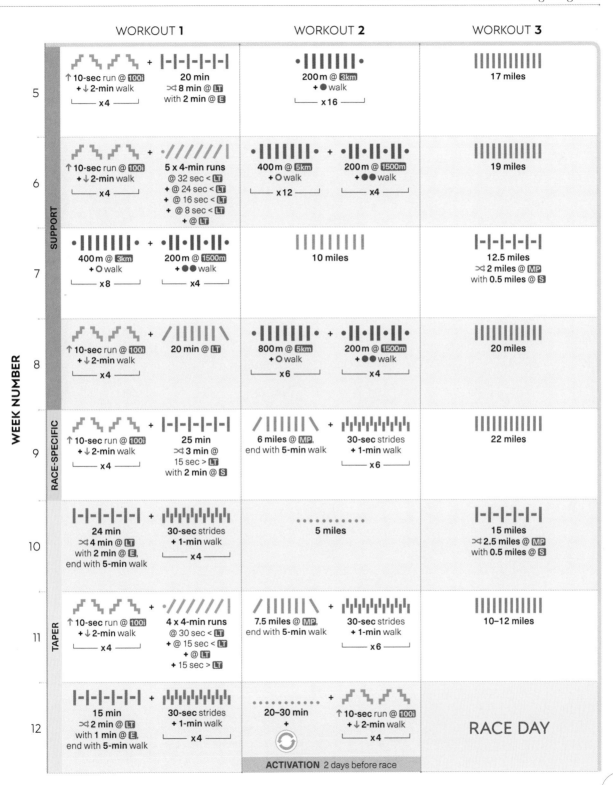

	WORKOUT **1**	WORKOUT **2**	WORKOUT **3**
5	↑ 10-sec run @ 100i + ↓ 2-min walk — x4 — + 20 min ⇄ 8 min @ LT with 2 min @ E	200 m @ 3km + ● walk — x16 —	17 miles
6	↑ 10-sec run @ 100i + ↓ 2-min walk — x4 — + 5 x 4-min runs @ 32 sec < LT + @ 24 sec < LT + @ 16 sec < LT + @ 8 sec < LT + @ LT	400 m @ 5km + ○ walk — x12 — + 200 m @ 1500m + ●● walk — x4 —	19 miles
7	400 m @ 3km + ○ walk — x8 — + 200 m @ 1500m + ●● walk — x4 —	10 miles	12.5 miles ⇄ 2 miles @ MP with 0.5 miles @ S
8	↑ 10-sec run @ 100i + ↓ 2-min walk — x4 — + 20 min @ LT	800 m @ 5km + ○ walk — x6 — + 200 m @ 1500m + ●● walk — x4 —	20 miles
9	↑ 10-sec run @ 100i + ↓ 2-min walk — x4 — + 25 min ⇄ 3 min @ 15 sec > LT with 2 min @ S	6 miles @ MP, end with 5-min walk + 30-sec strides + 1-min walk — x6 —	22 miles
10	24 min ⇄ 4 min @ LT with 2 min @ E, end with 5-min walk + 30-sec strides + 1-min walk — x4 —	5 miles	15 miles ⇄ 2.5 miles @ MP with 0.5 miles @ S
11	↑ 10-sec run @ 100i + ↓ 2-min walk — x4 — + 4 x 4-min runs @ 30 sec < LT + @ 15 sec < LT + @ LT + 15 sec > LT	7.5 miles @ MP, end with 5-min walk + 30-sec strides + 1-min walk — x6 —	10–12 miles
12	15 min ⇄ 2 min @ LT with 1 min @ E, end with 5-min walk + 30-sec strides + 1-min walk — x4 —	20–30 min + 🔄 + ↑ 10-sec run @ 100i + ↓ 2-min walk — x4 — **ACTIVATION** 2 days before race	**RACE DAY**

Column labels: SUPPORT (weeks 5–8), RACE-SPECIFIC (weeks 9–10), TAPER (weeks 11–12). Row axis: **WEEK NUMBER**

ADVANCED MARATHON PROGRAM

If you have completed a major race, this program is tailored to prepare you for the next one. Over the course of 24 weeks, it aims to improve your race time.

In this program, any workout that begins with marathon pace or faster (see pp.188–189) should be preceded by a 2-mile easy run and a dynamic warm-up.

INTRODUCTION PHASE

This phase helps you recover from the last major race. Build up to 60 percent of peak training volume with easy continuous runs and dynamic warm-ups before starting the next phase. This may take longer than three weeks, so repeat a week if needed.

BASE-BUILDING PHASE

Weeks 4–9 will increase aerobic volume, introduce aerobic intensity, and improve your running skills. Workout 1 introduces short sprints on hills and on the flat for interval training. Workout 2 consists of short to medium fast continuous runs that increase in intensity. The long runs of workout 3 become fast continuous runs that increase in volume and aerobic intensity.

SUPPORT PHASE

Recover in week 10 with lighter sessions for workouts 1 and 2. Weeks 11–15 aim to continue increasing aerobic volume and improve speed endurance, lactate threshold speed, and lactate clearance. In workout 1, VO_2 max intervals are introduced, recovery sections of the pace-change runs get faster, and hill runs become longer. In workout 2, the fast continuous runs become longer or faster in pace. Workout 3 increases the volume of the long runs, with more running at marathon pace.

RACE-SPECIFIC PHASE

This phase begins with lighter workouts in week 16 to aid recovery, then focuses on aerobic intensity with paces between marathon pace and slightly faster than lactate threshold (LT) pace. The short fast continuous runs of workout 1 focus on LT pace; for workout 2, the fast continuous runs get longer, becoming medium to long runs; while the workout 3 long fast continuous runs are at marathon goal pace. In weeks 17, 19, and 21, make sure you leave 2–3 days of recovery between marathon tempo runs for workout 2 and long runs for workout 3.

TAPER

The 3-week taper should kick-start recovery after the peak training weeks. Week 22, the initial taper, drops to 50 percent training volume; week 23 maintains your fitness with workouts that do not overly stress the body; and week 24 prevents sluggishness with a couple of easy workouts before your race day.

> **FOR KEY TO WORKOUT SYMBOLS SEE PP.188–189**

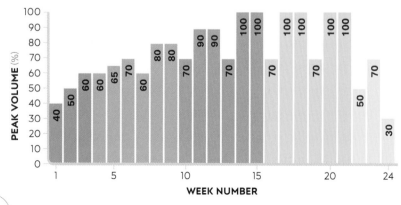

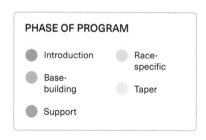

PHASE OF PROGRAM

- Introduction
- Base-building
- Support
- Race-specific
- Taper

TRAINING VOLUME PER WEEK
You will reach peak training volume by week 14, which is maintained (not increased) in the race-specific phase.

	WORKOUT **1**	WORKOUT **2**	WORKOUT **3**

WEEK NUMBER

INTRODUCTION

Week 1
- Workout 1: 30 min
- Workout 2: 30 min
- Workout 3: 8 miles

Week 2
- Workout 1: 40 min +
- Workout 2: 40 min +
- Workout 3: 9 miles

Week 3
- Workout 1: 60 min +
- Workout 2: 60 min +
- Workout 3: 10 miles

BASE-BUILDING

Week 4
- Workout 1: 30-sec sprint + 60–90-sec walk — x8
- Workout 2: 30 min — ⤨ 1 min @ 15 sec > **LT** with 2 min @ **E**
- Workout 3: 12 miles — ⤨ 3 miles @ **E** with 1 mile @ **MP**

Week 5
- Workout 1: ↑ 10-sec run @ **100!** + ↓ 2-min walk — x5 + 30-sec sprint + 60–90-sec walk — x5
- Workout 2: 30 min — 10 min @ 60 sec < **LT** + 8 min @ 45 sec < **LT** + 6 min @ 30 sec < **LT** + 4 min @ 15 sec < **LT** + 2 min @ **LT**
- Workout 3: 13 miles — 5 miles @ **E** + 3 miles @ 30 sec < **MP** + 5 miles @ **E**

Week 6
- Workout 1: ↑ 10-sec run @ **100!** + ↓ 2-min walk — x8 + 30-sec sprint + 60–90-sec walk — x4
- Workout 2: 50 min — 30 min @ **E** + 10 min @ **LT** + 10 min @ **E**
- Workout 3: 10 miles — 3 miles @ 60 sec < **MP** + 2.5 miles @ 45 sec < **MP** + 2 miles @ 30 sec < **MP** + 1.5 miles @ 15 sec < **MP** + 1 mile @ **MP**

Week 7
- Workout 1: ↑ 15-sec run @ **100!** + ↓ 2-min walk — x8 + 30-sec acceleration + 60–90-sec walk — x4
- Workout 2: 30 min — ⤨ 90 sec @ 15 sec > **LT** with 90 sec @ **E**
- Workout 3: 15 miles — ⤨ 4 miles @ **E** with 1 mile @ **MP**
  ***MP** sections can increase toward **LT** if you're feeling strong*

Week 8
- Workout 1: ↑ 15-sec run @ **100!** + ↓ 2-min walk — x10 + 30-sec acceleration + 60–90-sec walk — x4
- Workout 2: 5 x 6-min runs @ 60 sec < **LT** + @ 45 sec < **LT** + @ 30 sec < **LT** + @ 10 sec < **LT** + @ **LT**
- Workout 3: 9 miles — 3 miles @ **E** + 6 miles @ 30 sec < **MP**

MARATHON

ADVANCED

		WORKOUT 1	WORKOUT 2	WORKOUT 3
BASE-BUILDING	**9**	↑ 15-sec run @ 100i + ↓ 2-min walk — x10 — **+** 30-sec acceleration + 60–90-sec walk — x6 —	50 min 20 min @ E + 20 min @ LT + 10 min @ E	15 miles 7.5 miles @ 60 sec < MP + 5 miles @ 45 sec < MP + 2.5 miles @ 30 sec < MP
	10	30 min ⋈ 4 min @ LT with 2 min @ E	20–30 min + **+** ↑ 10-sec run @ 100i + ↓ 2-min walk — x4 — **ACTIVATION**	12 miles ⋈ 1 mile @ MP with 1 mile @ S *or substitute with 10 km race*
SUPPORT	**11**	↑ 15-sec run @ 100i + ↓ 2-min walk — x4 — ↑ 1-min run @ VO₂ + ↓ 2-min jog — x6 — **+** 1 min @ 3km + 1-min walk/ slow jog — x6 —	40 min ⋈ 6 min @ 15 sec > LT with 2 min @ E	16 miles 3 miles @ E + 10 miles @ 10 sec < MP + 3 miles @ E
	12	↑ 15-sec run @ 100i + ↓ 2-min walk — x4 — **+** 2 min @ 5km + 1-min walk/ slow jog — x10 —	30 min ⋈ 1 min @ 15 sec > LT with 2 min @ S	4 x 3-mile runs @ 72 sec < MP + @ 48 sec < MP + @ 24 sec < MP + @ MP
	13	↑ 15-sec run @ 100i + ↓ 2-min walk — x4 — **+** ↑ 90-sec run @ VO₂ + ↓ 3-min jog — x8 —	5 x 6-min runs @ 45 sec < LT + @ 30 sec < LT + @ 15 sec < LT + @ LT + @ 15 sec > LT	16 miles ⋈ 2 miles @ E with 2.5 miles, then 2 miles, then 1.5 miles, then 1 mile @ MP; end with 1 mile @ E
	14	↑ 15-sec run @ 100i + ↓ 2-min walk — x4 — **+** 3 min @ 5km + 90-sec walk/ slow jog — x6 —	48 min ⋈ 10 min @ 10 sec < LT with 2 min @ E	12 miles ⋈ 2 miles @ MP with 1 mile @ S
	15	↑ 15-sec run @ 100i + ↓ 2-min walk — x4 — ↑ 2-min run @ VO₂ + ↓ 4-min jog — x6 —	30 min ⋈ 90 sec @ 15 sec > LT with 90 sec @ S	19 miles 3 miles @ E + 13 miles @ 10 sec < MP + 3 miles @ E
RACE-SPECIFIC	**16**	30 min ⋈ 4 min @ LT with 2 min @ E	20–30 min + **+** ↑ 10-sec run @ 100i + ↓ 2-min walk — x4 — **ACTIVATION**	5 x 3-mile runs @ 60 sec < MP + @ 45 sec < MP + @ 30 sec < MP + @ 15 sec < MP + @ MP *or substitute with half marathon race*

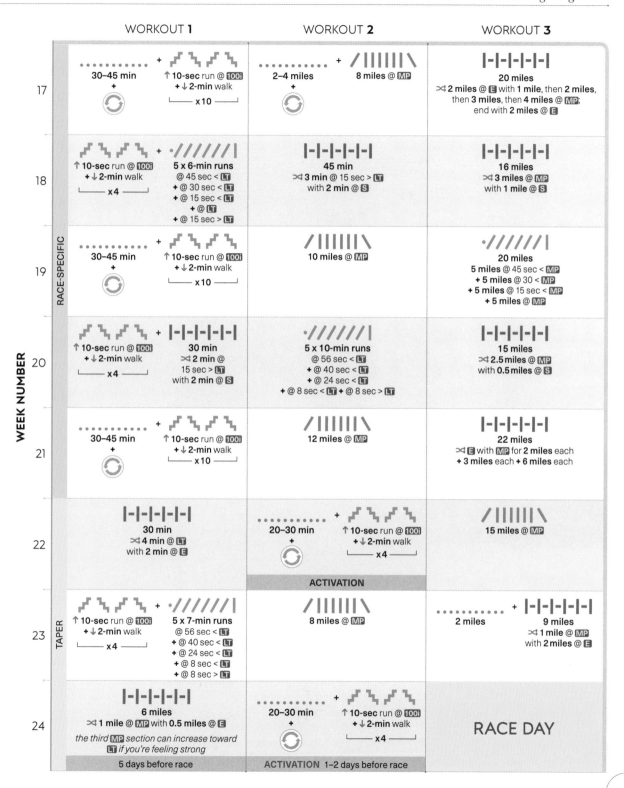

	WORKOUT **1**	WORKOUT **2**	WORKOUT **3**
17	30–45 min + ↻ ↑ 10-sec run @ 100i + ↓ 2-min walk — x10	2–4 miles + ↻ 8 miles @ MP	**20 miles** ⋈ 2 miles @ E with 1 mile, then 2 miles, then 3 miles, then 4 miles @ MP; end with 2 miles @ E
18	↑ 10-sec run @ 100i + ↓ 2-min walk — x4 5 x 6-min runs @ 45 sec < LT + @ 30 sec < LT + @ 15 sec < LT + @ LT + @ 15 sec > LT	**45 min** ⋈ 3 min @ 15 sec > LT with 2 min @ S	**16 miles** ⋈ 3 miles @ MP with 1 mile @ S
19	30–45 min + ↻ ↑ 10-sec run @ 100i + ↓ 2-min walk — x10	10 miles @ MP	**20 miles** 5 miles @ 45 sec < MP + 5 miles @ 30 < MP + 5 miles @ 15 sec < MP + 5 miles @ MP
20	↑ 10-sec run @ 100i + ↓ 2-min walk — x4 30 min ⋈ 2 min @ 15 sec > LT with 2 min @ S	5 x 10-min runs @ 56 sec < LT + @ 40 sec < LT + @ 24 sec < LT + @ 8 sec < LT + @ 8 sec > LT	**15 miles** ⋈ 2.5 miles @ MP with 0.5 miles @ S
21	30–45 min + ↻ ↑ 10-sec run @ 100i + ↓ 2-min walk — x10	12 miles @ MP	**22 miles** ⋈ E with MP for 2 miles each + 3 miles each + 6 miles each
22	30 min ⋈ 4 min @ LT with 2 min @ E	20–30 min + ↻ ↑ 10-sec run @ 100i + ↓ 2-min walk — x4 **ACTIVATION**	15 miles @ MP
23	↑ 10-sec run @ 100i + ↓ 2-min walk — x4 5 x 7-min runs @ 56 sec < LT + @ 40 sec < LT + @ 24 sec < LT + @ 8 sec < LT + @ 8 sec > LT	8 miles @ MP	2 miles + 9 miles ⋈ 1 mile @ MP with 2 miles @ E
24	**6 miles** ⋈ 1 mile @ MP with 0.5 miles @ E *the third MP section can increase toward LT if you're feeling strong* 5 days before race	20–30 min + ↻ ↑ 10-sec run @ 100i + ↓ 2-min walk — x4 **ACTIVATION** 1–2 days before race	**RACE DAY**

WEEK NUMBER

RACE-SPECIFIC (weeks 17–21)

TAPER (weeks 22–24)

RACING TIPS

Being prepared for race day will allow you to capitalize on all the hard work you have put in during training. Taking in the right fuel before the race, checking that your hydration levels are optimal, and putting a race strategy into action are all steps that can help you achieve your best.

> *Most people begin running for **health** and **fitness** but, once they **gain** **experience,** often want to **improve** their performance in **races***

NUTRITION

Ensuring you have proper fuel levels before and during the race is essential to power your body for the intense efforts ahead.

PRERACE CARB LOADING

In the days before a race, meals should be high in carbohydrates in order to build up stores of glycogen in your muscles. Your body will use this for fuel during the race.

For races longer than 90 minutes, have a big lunch the day before (about 18 hours before the race) to allow time to process the carbohydrates. Follow with a light dinner of simple carbohydrates and hydrate with a sports drink. Avoid high-fiber foods. For shorter races, eat a carbohydrate-filled dinner. If your race is not in the morning, eat light meals of simple carbohydrates throughout the day.

Top up glycogen stores with a small meal 2–3 hours before the race. If you experiment with optimal food and portion size in training, your prerace meal will not be new.

DURING THE RACE

Your body can store only a limited amount of fuel, and you will need to replenish during races that last longer than 90 minutes. Aim for approximately 2 oz (60 g) of carbohydrate intake per hour using easily absorbed sports drinks, gels, or similar foods. Determine your optimal intake during training (see box, below).

RACE SUPPLEMENTS

Legal performance-enhancing supplements may provide marginal gains but should never be a substitute for proper training and nutrition. For distance runners, caffeine and nitrate (found in beet juice) are two recommended supplements. However, test your tolerance of them during training, as they do not suit everyone.

Gut motility

Gastrointestinal complaints affect up to 70 percent of long-distance runners. During intense exercise, blood is directed away from your gut and toward your working muscles, which impairs your gut's ability to process food while you are running. Your gastrointestinal tract will be more able to absorb and process nutrition during a race if you have practiced taking on nutrition during your training sessions.

HYDRATION

How much you drink before and during a race will depend on environmental factors and the length and intensity of the race.

Drinking to thirst signals is better than overhydrating before and during the race. If you are well-hydrated (see hydration test, below)

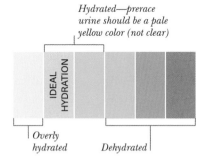

Hydrated—prerace urine should be a pale yellow color (not clear)

IDEAL HYDRATION

Overly hydrated

Dehydrated

and it is not a hot day, you should not need to drink much in the race. Many runners drink excessively, which can result in gastrointestinal issues and hyponatremia (see p.173). Ensure you replenish electrolytes lost through sweating during the race, and not just water. In longer races, fluid intake is often paired with fueling in the form of sports drinks. Experiment with how many and what type of calories you can absorb this way during training before trying it in a race.

HYDRATION TEST
Urine color is a good indicator of hydration. Use this color chart to assess your hydration levels before the race.

MUSCLE CRAMPING

Cramps are painful, involuntary muscle contractions that can incapacitate you if they happen during a race. Calf and foot cramps are the most common, but they also occur in hamstrings and quadriceps. New research refutes the traditional theory that cramps are caused by dehydration. Current theories suggest that fatiguing exercise causes sustained motor-neuron firing, resulting in cramps due to abnormal neuromuscular control. For immediate treatment, passively stretch the muscle (hold it in place or use the floor to maintain the stretch) until the cramping stops.

INVOLUNTARY CONTRACTION
A cramped calf muscle contracts suddenly and forcefully, causing the heel to plantarflex.

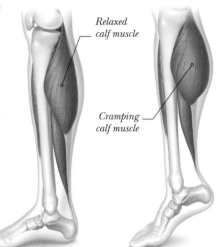

Relaxed calf muscle

Cramping calf muscle

Racing in a different time zone

If you are traveling to race in a time zone that is more than 3 hours different to your original time zone, jet lag can cause decreased performance. This can be more severe the more time zones you cross, if you travel in an easterly direction, if you are an older adult, or if you lack travel experience. The following tips can help your body clock synchronize with a new environment.

 Go for an easy jog shortly after arrival. This helps you acclimatize and wakes your brain up after the flight.

 Expose yourself to light at your destination, whether in the evening when traveling west to later time zones or in the morning when traveling east to an earlier time zone.

 Avoid light at your destination if you have traveled more than 8 time zones, either by wearing sunglasses until the late morning if traveling east or avoiding early evening sunlight if traveling west.

 Keep hydrated but avoid alcohol before and during the flight. Eat meals according to your destination's time zone to help your body clock adjust.

 Take short-acting sedatives to aid sleep, caffeine to keep you awake, or the sleep hormone melatonin to help you fight jet lag.

 Adjust your sleep schedule 1–2 days in advance of traveling. Go to bed 1–2 hours before your usual bedtime if traveling east or 1–2 hours later if traveling west.

RACE STRATEGY

Before your race, set some A, B, and C goals. Your A goal should be what you can achieve if all goes to plan and conditions are good. Your B goal should be a backup, and your C goal should be something that you can still be proud of if your race does not go according to plan.

The best way to ensure that you perform well on race day is to know what your body is capable of and how to pace appropriately. Of course, you will have learned these by following a structured training program. You should also have prepared for the terrain, for example, by doing hill training to gear up for a hilly course.

However, unpredictable weather conditions or terrain may prevent you from following your plan. If this is the case, adjust your race strategy to suit the course and conditions so that you run by effort (in other words, by what you know your goal pace feels like) rather than continuing to hold onto a predetermined pace.

Why you may race faster than you train

If you have prepared well and tapered your training effectively, you should reach race day well rested and in an energy-rich state.

Heightened feelings of excitement on race day cause the sympathetic nervous system's "fight-or-flight" response (see p.42) to release a surge of adrenaline, which allows your body to perform at a higher level than in training. The simple motivation of it being a race and not just another workout can also have a dramatic effect on your performance.

Planning your race

One useful strategy is to divide the race into four phases: Pace, Position, Drive, Kick. Each phase has a goal that you can match to your overall plan. You may decide to pace yourself evenly or to start slower and increase pace later. This will depend on the terrain, conditions, and belief in your ability to hold a chosen pace.

RACE BREAKDOWN
Split your race distance into stages at which you can implement your strategy. Divide the first three phases equally, but the final "Kick" should be saved for the last stretch.

PACE

AIM: *Settle into your planned pace*

- **Have in mind a starting pace** (or effort) that you know you can sustain.

- **At the starting line**, it is easy to get swept up in the excitement and start too fast. This can interfere with your pacing early in the race, so it is important to stay calm, run your own race, and settle into your pace.

- **Get comfortable** at your planned pace and monitor how your perceived effort is matching up with your planned pace. Try not to pay too much attention to what is going on around you.

POSITION

AIM: *Find a good position for your strategy*

- **Look around you.** If there are people running at your pace, latch onto a group to reduce the mental burden and share the pacemaking.

- **If your goal is to win** or place well, play to your strengths. Runners with good speed may choose to "sit and kick" by staying behind the leader and speeding past them at the end. A runner with good endurance may choose to lead and increase the pace, exhausting other competitors until they cannot keep up.

5 KM		
1.5 KM		1.5–3 KM
10 KM		
3.5 KM		3.5–6.5 KM
HALF MARATHON		
7 KM		7–14 KM
MARATHON		
14 KM		14–28 KM

Race recovery

Competing in a race takes maximal effort, and you should plan to take a couple of days to a couple of weeks off training to recover, depending on the length and intensity of the race. Your recovery should be active, but make sure your activities are low in impact and intensity (see p.174).

The training program leading up to a race, especially a marathon, can take its toll both mentally and physically. Take care of any ailments that may have cropped up during the build-up or in the race. Use this time to catch up on work, social engagements, and other things that may have taken a back seat in your life while you focused on race preparations. Most importantly, make sure you reward yourself for all the hard work you have put in and what you have achieved.

Deciding when to return to training will depend on how your body is feeling in the aftermath of the race. You should start with easy continuous running until you feel your legs have recovered, then add some strides or short sprints to your workouts to activate your neuromuscular system. Build this recovery time into your seasonal plan (see p.161).

Racing highs and lows

Your body can react to the exertion of racing in extreme ways. You may be lucky, or unlucky, enough to experience these two phenomena.

Runners' high, a feeling of euphoria induced by long-distance running, is a legend told by runners around the world. Until recently, there was little science to explain this phenomenon. Now, advances in brain imaging can verify that endurance running sets off a flood of hormones in the brain. Known as endorphins, these hormones are associated with mood uplift and elation. This endorphin release appears to be an example of a neurological "reward" response to intense aerobic activity, which is likely part of our evolutionary history.

The "wall" is a physiological state caused by depleting glycogen stores in the liver and muscles. When this happens, you may feel sudden and extreme fatigue, heaviness, loss of coordination in the legs, blurry vision, and a lack of concentration. Most marathon runners can relate to "hitting the wall" in the later stages of a race. While the condition can be mitigated by adequate fueling (see p.210) and pacing, recent research suggests that your physiology and metabolism actually change after approximately 90 minutes of running, making what seemed to you like a sustainable pace now difficult to maintain.

DRIVE

AIM: *Maintain your plan and set yourself up for a big finish*

- **As you fatigue**, focusing on relaxation signals and practicing self-talk can help get you through those tough moments when you want to quit.

- **Dig deep** into your energy reserves and increase your pace—if you are able to—or at least maintain your pace. Push yourself for a personal best or top placing.

KICK

AIM: *Finish as fast as possible*

- **Use that last rush** of adrenaline and motivation to sprint for the finish line.

- **Prepare to accelerate** when you reach the last 500 m of the race. In a shorter race, you may be able to "kick" up the pace for up to 400 m. At the end of a marathon, you may only be able to sprint the last 100 m.

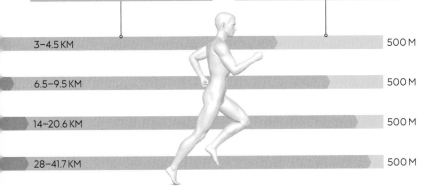

3–4.5 KM	500 M
6.5–9.5 KM	500 M
14–20.6 KM	500 M
28–41.7 KM	500 M

GLOSSARY

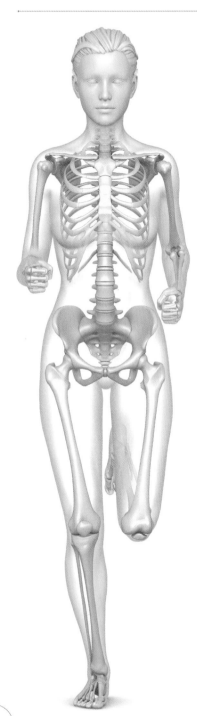

adenosine triphosphate (ATP) The molecule that stores, transports, and releases the energy used to power muscle contractions.

aerobic respiration The primary method of energy production during endurance exercise, when the body uses oxygen to convert glucose into ATP.

alactic The most immediately available energy system, it powers sudden or explosive movements. The anaerobic alactic system is fueled by stored ATP and creatine phosphate.

anaerobic respiration The method of energy production the body uses during strenuous exercise when there is a shortage of oxygen. Results in lactate accumulation, so it can only last a short time.

biomechanics The study of forces and movements of the body during running—also known as "running form."

concentric A type of muscle contraction during which the muscle is shortened.

distal Bodily structures situated farther away from the core of the body.

early loading phase The beginning of the running cycle; involves the first 15–20 percent of stance as the leading foot makes initial contact with the ground.

eccentric A type of muscle contraction during which the muscle lengthens.

external load An objective measure of the volume of work done by the body, such as distance, time, or steps taken.

float phase The period of time in running during which both feet are off the ground. This is a subphase of the swing phase in the running cycle and is also known as "flight phase."

footstrike pattern The location on the foot that first makes contact with the ground. Footstrike patterns are classified as rearfoot, midfoot, or forefoot.

goal pace The estimated pace in minutes per mile or kilometer you must run to achieve a goal race time.

ground reaction force (GRF) The equal and opposite force applied to the body during contact with the ground.

heart rate reserve (HRR) The range of heart activity available to you for exercise; the difference between your resting heart rate (RHR) and your maximum heart rate.

internal load The measure of effort you put in during a workout or race, such as heart rate, breathing rate, or RPE.

isometric A type of muscle contraction during which the muscle does not change in length.

kinematics The measurement of motion of the human body without respect to forces (for example, joint angles).

kinetic chain A concept that describes the body as a chain of linked segments. Each segment contributes individual movements that link up with adjoining segments into larger movements along the chain.

kinetic energy Energy created by motion.

lactate threshold The highest intensity of exercise you can manage before your body begins to exponentially accumulate lactate.

midstance phase The period during which the center of mass (COM) is directly over the top of the base of support, when the maximum vertical GRF occurs and the braking force transitions to a propulsive force.

moment or torque A measure of how much a force acting on an object causes that object to rotate about an axis.

PB Personal best.

proximal Bodily structures situated closer to the core of the body.

rate of perceived exertion (RPE) scale
A quantitative measure of the effort imparted during exercise. RPE is measured on an 11-point scale.

running economy The energy demand for a given velocity of submaximal running, determined by measuring the steady-state consumption of oxygen (VO₂) and the respiratory exchange ratio. Variables such as genetics, environmental conditions, running shoes, fitness, and biomechanics can affect the amount of oxygen used at a given speed.

running form *see* biomechanics

stance phase The period during which the foot is in contact with the ground when running. It comprises approximately 40 percent of the running cycle (less as speed increases).

swing phase The period of running during which the foot is not in contact with the ground. It comprises approximately 60 percent of the running cycle (more with increasing speed).

terminal stance phase The final subphase of the stance phase when the hip, knee, and ankle are in maximal extension to propel the body forward.

toe-off The moment the foot leaves the ground to drive the body forward.

training load An overall measure of stress on the body due to training. This is calculated as the product of the volume (external load) and intensity (internal load) of your workouts.

training volume The measure of the quantity and effort involved in training, often measured in miles, kilometers, or by duration.

VO₂ max A measure of how much oxygen the body can consume during maximal effort.

MUSCLE GROUPS

deep six muscles A group of hip external rotator muscles that is commonly tight in distance runners.

distal hamstrings The end of the hamstring muscles closest to the knee. Their action is to flex the knee.

external rotators (of the hip) Muscles that rotate the hip outward.

hip abductors Muscles that help maintain pelvic stability in the frontal plane during running. Hip abductors resist contralateral pelvic drop.

hip adductors Muscle group on the inside of the thigh that pulls the thigh in toward the midline. Includes adductor longus, adductor brevis, adductor magnus, pectineus, and gracilis.

hip extensors Muscle group that extends the hip and draws the thigh back. Includes gluteals, adductor magnus, and hamstrings.

hip flexors Muscle group that flexes the hip and raises the thigh up toward the chest. Includes iliopsoas (iliacus and psoas major), rectus femoris, sartorius, and tensor fasciae latae (TFL).

internal rotators (of the hip) Muscles that rotate the hip inward.

proximal hamstrings The end of the hamstring muscles closest to the hip. Proximal hamstrings extend the hip.

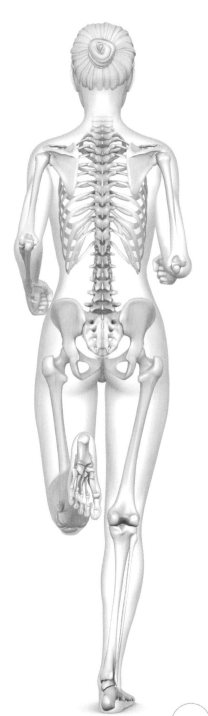

INDEX

BIBLIOGRAPHY

INTRODUCTION

6 *"Running has one of the highest participation rates of any sport."* M. van Middelkoop et al., "Risk factors for lower extremity injuries among male marathon runners," Scand J Med Sci Sports 18 (2008). *"Even in low doses, running is associated with a substantial reduction in cardiovascular disease."* C. J. Lavie et al., "Exercise and the cardiovascular system," AHA Circulation Research 117 (2015).

8 *"If you have osteoarthritis, running may not make it worse and could in fact improve symptoms."* G. H. Lo et al., "Running does not increase symptoms or structural progression in people with knee osteoarthritis," Clinical Rheumatology 37 (2018).

9 *"A heavy resistance training program twice a week for 6 weeks or longer has been shown to improve running performance and reduce injury risk."* J. B. Lauersen et al., "The effectiveness of exercise interventions to prevent sports injuries," British Journal of Sports Medicine 48 (2014).

RUNNING ANATOMY

24 *"A larger Q-angle has been associated with an increased injury risk, and in particular to patellofemoral pain, but research does not support this link."* G .P. Almeida et al., "Q-angle in patellofemoral pain: relationship with dynamic knee valgus, hip abductor torque, pain, and function," Revista Brasileira de Ortopedia 51 (2016). N. E. Lankhorst, S. M. Bierma-Zeinstra, M. van Middelkoop, "Risk factors for patellofemoral pain syndrome," Journal of Orthopedic & Sports Physical Therapy 42 (2012). E. Pappas, W. M. Wong-Tom, "Prospective predictors of patellofemoral pain syndrome," Sports Health 4 (2012).

30 *"A well-functioning core allows you to control your trunk over your planted leg, maximizing the production, transfer, and control of force and motion to your lower limbs."* W. B. Kibler et al., "The role of core stability in athletic function," Sports Medicine 36 (2006).

31 *"Running has been shown to improve the health of the intervertebral discs."* D. L. Belavy et al., "Running exercise strengthens the intervertebral disc," Scientific Reports 7 (2017).

46 *"Some studies have linked the vertical GRF loading rate with injury, while others have found associations between injury and the braking (anterior-posterior) force."* H. van der Worp et al., "Do runners who suffer injuries have higher vertical ground reaction forces than those who remain injury-free?", British Journal of Sports Medicine 50 (2016). C. Napier et al., "Kinetic risk factors of running-related injuries in female recreational runners," Scand J Med Sci Sports 28 (2018).

50 *"As little as 10 days training in the heat has been shown to boost VO₂ max values by 5 percent."* S. Lorenzo et al., "Heat acclimation improves exercise performance," Journal of Applied Physiology 109 (2010). *"Running economy improves while drafting behind someone, especially when running into a headwind."* I. Shinichiro, "Aerodynamic Effects by Marathon Pacemakers on a Main Runner," Transactions of the Japan Society of Mechanical Engineers, Part B 73 (2007). C. T. Davies, "Effects of wind assistance and resistance on the forward motion of a runner," Journal of applied physiology: respiratory, environmental, and exercise physiology 48 (1980).

51 *"Even exposure to high levels of traffic-related pollution does not outweigh the beneficial effects of physical activity."* Z. J. Andersen, A. de Nazelle, M. A. Mendez et al., "A study of the combined effects of physical activity and air pollution on mortality in elderly urban residents," Environmental Health Perspectives 123 (2015).

PREVENTING INJURY

54 *"Improving your running form may help to protect against injury."* Z. Y. S. Chan, J. H. Zhang, I. P. H. Au et al., "Gait Retraining for the Reduction of Injury Occurrence in Novice Distance Runners: 1-Year Follow-up of a Randomized Controlled Trial," American Journal of Sports Medicine 46 (2018).

64 *"Stride parameters and footstrike patterns remained unchanged after a 6-month transition to minimalist footwear … there are also conflicting findings on the effect of minimalist shoes on loading rates."* J. T. Fuller, D. Thewlis, MD Tsiros et al., "Longer-term effects of minimalist shoes on running performance, strength, and bone density: a 20-week follow-up study," European Journal of Sport Science (2018). J. P. Warne, A. H. Gruber AH, "Transitioning to minimal footwear: a systematic review of methods and future clinical recommendations," Sports Medicine 3 (2017).

65 *"Females are more prone to knee injuries and males suffer more ankle, foot, and shin injuries."* P. Francis, C. Whatman, K. Sheerin K et al., "The Proportion of Lower Limb Running Injuries by Gender, Anatomical Location, and Specific Pathology," Journal of Sports Science and Medicine 18 (2019).

72 *"The notions that a rearfoot strike increases injury risk and that a forefoot strike is more economical have both been refuted by recent research."* J. Hamill and A. H. Gruber, "Is changing footstrike pattern beneficial to runners?", J Sport Health Sci 6 (2017).

73 *"Contralateral pelvic drop was the most important variable for running-related injuries."* C. Bramah C, S. J. Preece, N. Gill et al., "Is There a Pathological Gait Associated with Common Soft Tissue Running Injuries?", American Journal of Sports Medicine 46 (2018).

STRENGTH EXERCISES
97 *"Strength training has a beneficial effect not just on injury risk, but also on performance."* B. R. Rønnestad et al., "Optimizing strength training for running and cycling endurance performance," Scand J Med Sci Sports 24 (2014).

102 *"The foot provides up to 17 percent of the energy required to power a stride."* L. A. Kelly et al., "Intrinsic foot muscles contribute to elastic energy storage and return in the human foot," Journal of Applied Physiology 126 (2019).

116 *"Approximately one in five people with acute ankle sprains go on to develop chronic ankle instability."* O. A. Al-Mohrej et al., "Chronic ankle instability: Current perspectives," Avicenna Journal of Medicine 6 (2016).

128 *"The degree of anterior pelvic tilt during running affects the amount of hip extension achieved in toe-off."* A. G. Schache et al., "Relation of anterior pelvic tilt during running to clinical and kinematic measures of hip extension," British Journal of Sports Medicine 34 (2000).

152 *"Long-distance running does not decrease the risk for stress fracture."* P. Mustajoki et al., "Calcium metabolism, physical activity, and stress fractures," The Lancet 322 (1983).
A. Swissa et al., "The effect of pretraining sports activity on the incidence of stress fractures among military recruits," Clinical Orthopedics and Related Research 245 (1989).
M. Fredericson, J. Ngo, and K. Cobb, "Effects of ball sports on future risk of stress fractures in runners," Clinical Journal of Sports Medicine 15 (2005).
"Exercises that rapidly subject the body to high loads, such as hopping or jumping off a box, are recommended to stiffen bone and reduce stress fracture risk." C. Milgrom et al., "Using Bone's Adaptation Ability to Lower the Incidence of Stress Fractures," American Journal of Sports Medicine 28 (2000).

HOW TO TRAIN
168 *"Lactate threshold can be measured in a lab, but another simple way is to use the RPE scale."* J. L. Dantas et al., "Detection of the lactate threshold in runners: what is the ideal speed to start an incremental test?", Journal of Human Kinetics 45 (2015).

170 *"Listening to fast-paced music can help push your body further while your brain is occupied."* J. Waterhouse, P. Hudson, B. Edwards, "Effects of music tempo upon submaximal cycling performance," Scand J Med Sci Sports 20 (2010).

171 *"When things get tough, telling yourself "I can do this" or "I can work through the pain" can improve your race performance."* A. W. Blanchfield, J. Hardy, H. M. De Morree et al., "Talking yourself out of exhaustion: the effects of self-talk on endurance performance," Medicine & Science in Sports & Exercise 46 (2014).

175 *"Although evidence suggests that it does not increase blood flow or help with removal of metabolic waste products (both often said to be benefits of massage), the positive psychological effects of massage are consistently reported in scientific studies."* O. Dupuy et al., "An Evidence-Based Approach for Choosing Post-exercise Recovery Techniques to Reduce Markers of Muscle Damage, Soreness, Fatigue, and Inflammation," Frontiers in Physiology (2018).
"Proper sleep hygiene can enhance sleep quality and quantity." S. L. Halson et al., "Monitoring training load to understand fatigue in athletes," Sports Medicine 44 (2014).

182 *"Physiologically, these workouts increase the oxygen uptake in a higher percentage of muscle fibers, accelerating turnover by engaging first the slow-twitch muscle fibers and then the fast-twitch fibers in the later stages of the run."* R. Canova, Marathon Training: A Scientific Approach, IAF, 1999 (p.51).

183 *"The slow-twitch muscles that are activated in the slower sections clear the lactate build-up, improving your muscles' ability to use lactate as fuel."* R. Canova, Marathon Training: A Scientific Approach, IAF, 1999 (p.53).
"Being able to keep the pace of the recoveries as close to the fast pace as possible, or to decrease their duration, indicates that your muscles have improved ability to clear lactate." R. Canova, Marathon Training: A Scientific Approach, IAF, 1999 (p.52).

185 *"Marathoners with fast 5 km and 10 km race times will be better served with training that is closer to lactate threshold."* R. Canova, Marathon Training: A Scientific Approach, IAF, 1999 (pp.60–62).

210 *"Gastrointestinal complaints affect up to 70 percent of long-distance runners."* H. P. Peters et al., "Gastrointestinal symptoms in long-distance runners, cyclists, and triathletes: prevalence, medication, and etiology," The American Journal of Gastroenterology 96 (1999).

211 *"Drinking to thirst is still your best strategy rather than overhydrating before and during your race."* E. D. B. Goulet, MD. Hoffman, "Impact of Ad Libitum Versus Programmed Drinking on Endurance Performance," Sports Medicine 49 (2019).

213 *"Physiology and metabolism change after approximately 90 minutes of running."* I. E. Clark et al., "Dynamics of the power-duration relationship during prolonged endurance exercise and influence of carbohydrate ingestion," Journal of Applied Physiology 127 (2019).

ABOUT THE AUTHORS

Chris Napier is a clinician, a researcher specialising in running injury prevention, and a keen runner. He is co-owner of Restore Physiotherapy, a private practice in Vancouver, Canada, and a Clinical Assistant Professor in the Department of Physical Therapy at the University of British Columbia (UBC). He is a physical therapist with Athletics Canada, and has worked with Commonwealth, Pan Am, Olympic, and World Championship teams. As a runner, he earned a silver medal at the Canadian Junior Track & Field Championships in 1996 and a bronze medal at the Canadian University Track & Field Championships in 1997 in the middle distances. Having moved up to the marathon in 2010, he has enjoyed chipping away at his personal best over the years with the help of his coach and co-author, Jerry Ziak.

Jerry Ziak has been a competitive distance runner since 1986, a coach since 2005, and co-owner of the running specialty store Forerunners North Shore, Vancouver, since 2013. His competitive running career began over cross-country and on the track, where he specialized in middle distances ranging from 800 m to 10,000 m. He ran for Auburn University in Alabama, Boise State University in Idaho, and the University of Victoria in British Columbia before settling down at the University of British Columbia. He used this varied experience to self-coach himself over longer distances, ultimately achieving a time of 2:17:24 for the marathon. He also began to coach high school cross-country and track, as well as half marathon and marathon clinics. He continues to compete over a range of distances into his forties and enjoys sharing his knowledge and passion for the sport via his store, his running clinics, and online coaching.

ACKNOWLEDGMENTS

Authors' acknowledgments

Chris: I owe a great deal of thanks to many people in my life for making this book possible. To Kate, Bella, and Roewan for your continual support. To my mother, who still inspires me by winning her age group, and to my late father, who first advised me on the "sit and kick" strategy. To my many coaches over the years— especially my co-author and friend, Jerry Ziak—whom I have learned from immensely. To my friends and peers—Paul Blazey, Lara Boyd, and Tara Klassen—who helped in proofreading, editing, and advising. And to the editorial team at DK, who were an absolute pleasure to work with: Salima, Alastair, Clare, Tia, Arran, and many more.

Jerry: I would like to thank my family for their ongoing support of my passion for running. I am also indebted to all my former coaches and particularly to my childhood coach and lifelong friend, Darren Skuja, who ignited my love for the sport at a young age.

Publisher's acknowledgments: DK would like to thank Mark Lloyd and Karen Constanti for additional design, Constance Novis for proofreading, and Ruth Ellis for indexing.

Picture credits: The publisher would like to thank the following for their kind permission to reproduce their photographs:
(Key: a-above; b-below/bottom; c-center; f-far; l-left; r-right; t-top)

16 Science Photo Library: Professors P.M. Motta, P.M. Andrews, K.R. Porter & J. Vial (clb). **27 Stuart Hinds**: Based the figure "Types of FAI (Femoral Acetabular Impingement)" (br). **32 Science Photo Library**: Steve Gschmeissner (cb); Professor P.M. Motta & E. Vizza (crb). **33 Science Photo Library**: Professors P. Motta & T. Naguro (clb). **34 Science Photo Library**: CNRI (cla); Ikelos Gmbh / Dr. Christopher B. Jackson (clb). **35 Based on fig.7 from Introduction to Exercise Science by Stanley P. Brown (Lippincott Williams and Wilkins, 2000)**: (bl). **50 Practically Science**: Based on a figure by Eugene Douglass and Chad Miller from "The Science of Drafting" (bl). **51 The Conversation**: Based on The Impact of altitude on oxygen levels graph by Brendan Scott (b). **55 Journal of Sports Science and Medicine**: Based on fig. 2, 3 and 4 from "The Proportion of Lower Limb Running Injuries by Gender, Anatomical Location and Specific Pathology: A Systematic Review." Francis, Peter et al. Journal of sports science & medicine vol. 18,1 21–31. 11 Feb. 2019 (r/graph). **72 Springer Nature**: Based on fig. 1(a) and 1(c) from Foot strike patterns and collision forces in habitually barefoot versus shod runners. Lieberman DE, Venkadesan M, Werbel WA, Daoud AI, D'Andrea S, Davis IS, Mang'eni RO & Pitsiladis Y. Nature 463, 531-535 (2010), DOI: 10.1038/nature08723 (b). **147 Data based on fig. from Clinical Biomechanics of the Spine by A. A. White and M. M. Panjabi (Philadelphia: Lippincott, 1978)**: (t). **159 © The Running Clinic**: Based on a diagram by The Running Clinic (t). **164 McMillan Running**: data generated by McMillan Running Calculator - mcmillanrunning. com. **170–171 Springer Science and Bus Media B V**: Based on fig.1 in "Do we really need a central governor to explain brain regulation of exercise performance?" Marcora, Samuele (2008). European journal of applied physiology. 104. 929-31; author reply 933. DOI: 10.1007/s00421-008-0818-3. / Copyright Clearance Center - Rightslink (b). **172 University of Colorado Colorado Springs**: Based on The Athlete's Plates developed by Meyer, NL with UCCS' Sport Nutrition Graduate Program in collaboration with the US Olympic Committee's (USOC) Food and Nutrition Services (b).

All other images © **Dorling Kindersley**
For further information see: **www.dkimages.com**